MRCPsych Paper 2

600 MCQs

Ashok G Patel MBBS DPM FRCPsych
Consultant General Adult Psychiatrist (Retired)
South Essex Partnership University NHS Foundation Trust
Luton, UK

Samir Shah MBBS MRCPsych MSc
Consultant Psychiatrist in General Adult Psychiatry
Cheshire and Wirral Partnership NHS Foundation Trust
Macclesfield, UK

Syed Ashraf MBBS PGCHM
Specialty Doctor in Psychiatry
South Essex Partnership University NHS Foundation Trust
Bedford Hospital
Bedford, UK

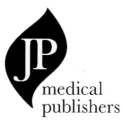

JP
medical
publishers

London • Philadelphia • Panama City • New Delhi

© 2014 JP Medical Ltd.
Published by JP Medical Ltd,
83 Victoria Street, London, SW1H 0HW, UK
Tel: +44 (0)20 3170 8910
Fax: +44 (0)20 3008 6180
Email: info@jpmedpub.com
Web: www.jpmedpub.com

ISBN: 978-1-907816-40-6

British Library Cataloguing in Publication Data
A catalogue record for this book is available from the British Library

Library of Congress Cataloging in Publication Data
A catalog record for this book is available from the Library of Congress

JP Medical Ltd is a subsidiary of Jaypee Brothers Medical Publishers (P) Ltd, New Delhi, India

Commissioning Editor: Steffan Clements
Design: Designers Collective Ltd

Typeset, printed and bound in India.

Preface

The MRCPsych examinations are extremely challenging, and candidates must be meticulous in their preparation if they are to stand any chance of success. Understanding this principle has been fundamental during our preparation of this book, and we have endeavoured to provide sufficient MCQ revision material for each element of the curriculum. We are confident that by using this book, readers will be well armed to face the MCQ component of the Paper 2 exam.

In order to facilitate revision, we have mapped the questions in the first four chapters to the curriculum topics. The fifth chapter is intentionally unstructured, and has been included to provide a mock exam representative of the MCQ component of Paper 2, which readers can use to practise under exam conditions. All questions are based on the curriculum and thorough answers have been provided to explain the rationale behind each correct answer option.

The burden of editorship has been wisely spread to harness varied expertise. In psychiatry, innovation in practice tends to be evolutionary rather than revolutionary, and much of our knowledge remains to be translated into practical innovations in patient care. It is our intention that this book will help psychiatry trainees not only to pass the MRCPsych Paper 2 examination, but also to improve their patient care. We believe that the book will assist trainees, trainers, educational and clinical supervisors, College tutors, Directors of Medical Education, SAS tutors and Training Programme Directors in preparation for the MRCPsych examinations.

Ashok G Patel
Samir Shah
Syed Ashraf
December 2013

Contents

Acknowledgements

We would like to thank the colleagues and friends who have helped us as we prepared this book. They have been a great source of useful advice and suggestions and have read the draft papers to make sure that the questions and answers were compatible with the MRCPsych Paper 2 exam.

We are also most grateful to the many people behind the scenes without whose help this book would not have been possible. In particular, we would like to thank the publishers, especially Steffan Clements, Hannah Applin and Katrina Rimmer for their encouragement and support from the very beginning to the end of the project. Special thanks go to Sue Keely and Mrs Vasanthi Varadharajan in preparing the manuscripts.

We would like to thank Nicola Cowdery, Deepak Garg, Vineel Reddy, Khurram Sadiq, Ajaya Upadhyaya, Dinesh Khanna, Faisal Pervez, Sanjith Kamath, Vishelle Kamath, Basavaraja Papanna and Juhi Mishra for their support and encouragement.

Finally, we would also like to thank the families of the authors and our own families for putting up with us as inevitably the book has been written during evenings, weekends and holidays.

AP, SS, SA

Contributing Authors

Syed Ashraf MBBS PGCHM
Chapter 1: Questions and Answers
Specialty Doctor in Psychiatry
South Essex Partnership University NHS
Foundation Trust
Bedford Hospital
Bedford, UK

Gursharan Lal Kashyap MBBS DCH MD
MRCPsych
Chapter 1: Questions and Answers
Specialist Registrar Year 5 in Psychiatry
South Essex Partnership University NHS
Foundation Trust
Bedford Hospital
Bedford, UK

Sanjith Kamath MBBS MRCPsych
Chapter 5: Questions and Answers
Consultant General Adult Psychiatrist
St Andrews Healthcare
Northampton, UK

Vishelle Kamath MBBS MRCPsych
Chapter 5: Questions and Answers
Consultant Old Age Psychiatrist
South Essex Partnership University NHS
Foundation Trust
Houghton Regis, UK

Dinesh Khanna MBBS MSc MRCPsych
Chapter 2: Questions and Answers
Specialty Trainee Year 6 in Child and Adolescent
Mental Health Services
Greater Manchester West Mental Health NHS
Foundation Trust
Prestwich Hospital
Manchester, UK

Faisal Parvez MBBS MRCPsych
Chapter 4: Questions and Answers
Specialist Registrar Year 6 in Old Age Psychiatry
The Meadows Community Hospital
Stockport NHS Foundation Trust
Offerton, UK

Roshelle Ramkisson MBBS MRCPsych MSC
(Health and Public Leadership) PGDip
Psychiatry MDCH
Chapter 2: Questions and Answers
Consultant Psychiatrist in Child and Adolescent
Psychiatry
Pennine Care NHS Foundation Trust
Royal Oldham Hospital
Oldham, UK

Madhavan Seshadri MBBS DPM MRCPsych
Chapter 3: Questions and Answers
Specialist Registrar Year 6 in Psychiatry
South Essex Partnership University NHS
Foundation Trust
Bedford Hospital
Bedford, UK

Raman Sharma MBBS MSc (Psychiatric Practice)
MRCPsych
Chapter 3: Questions and Answers
Specialty Doctor in Psychiatry
South Essex Partnership University NHS
Foundation Trust
Bedford Hospital
Bedford, UK

Ankush Singhal MBBS MD MRCPsych
Chapter 4: Questions and Answers
Consultant Liaison Psychiatrist
Pennine Care NHS Foundation Trust
The Royal Oldham Hospital,
Oldham, UK

Chapter 1

Test questions: 1

Questions: MCQs

For each question, select one answer option.

NEUROSCIENCES: NEUROANATOMY

1. Which of the following is the commonest neuroglia found in the peripheral nervous system?

   A   Astrocytes
   B   Ependymal cells
   C   Microglia
   D   Oligodendrocytes
   E   Schwann cells

2. A 45-year-old woman was diagnosed with an intrinsic brain tumour. Which of the following is the most likely tumour?

   A   Chordoma
   B   Epidermoid
   C   Meningioma
   D   Neuroma
   E   Oligodendroglioma

3. Which of the following brain structures include a dentate nucleus?

   A   Cerebral hemisphere
   B   Cerebellum
   C   Medulla oblongata
   D   Midbrain
   E   Pons

4. Astereognosis is the inability to recognise objects by touching and is linked to Brodmann's areas. Which of the following Brodmann's areas are affected in a stereognosis?

   A   5, 7
   B   8, 9
   C   9, 10
   D   18, 19, 20
   E   22, 42

5. Which of the following is most likely to be due to a lesion in left Brodmann's areas 39 and 40?

   A   Acalculia
   B   Agraphia without alexia
   C   Alexia with agraphia
   D   Alexia without agraphia
   E   Gerstmann's syndrome

NEUROSCIENCES: NEUROPATHOLOGY

6.   Which of the following about the neuropathology of schizophrenia is correct?

   A   Increase in temporal lobe volume
   B   No reduction in the anteroposterior length of the cerebral hemisphere
   C   Parahippocampal gyrus is significantly smaller
   D   Significant differences found in hippocampal area
   E   Slight and insignificant reduction in brain mass

7.   Which of the following are characteristic changes seen in patients with the punch-drunk syndrome?

   A   Cerebral hypertrophy
   B   Neuronal hyperplasia
   C   Perforation of the septum pellucidum
   D   Thickening of the corpus callosum
   E   Ventricular shrinkage

8.   A 72-year-old man was diagnosed with Alzheimer's disease. Which of the following brain regions sustain most atrophy change?

   A   Basal ganglia
   B   Cerebellum
   C   Locus ceruleus
   D   Substantia nigra
   E   Temporal lobe

9.   A 42-year-old man was diagnosed with Pick's disease. Which of the following pathological features is most likely to be found?

   A   Global brain atrophy
   B   Knife blade gyri
   C   Sulcal widening
   D   Symmetrical atrophy of the anterior temporal lobes
   E   Ventricular shrinkage

10. Which of the following is the characteristic pathological feature of Creutzfeldt–Jakob disease?

   A   Generalised cerebral atrophy
   B   Neurofibrillary tangles
   C   Neuritic plaques
   D   Neuronal loss
   E   Ventricular shrinkage

NEUROSCIENCES: NEUROPHYSIOLOGY

11. Which of the following regulates growth hormone from the anterior pituitary gland?

   A   Combined growth hormone-releasing hormone (GHRH) and somatostatins
   B   GHRH
   C   Prolactin
   D   Somatostatins
   E   Thyroid-stimulating hormone

12. Which of the following is a ligand-gated channel?

    A   Calcium channels
    B   Calcium-activated potassium channel
    C   Glutamate receptors
    D Na^+ channels
    E   Potassium channels

13. Each electroencephalogram (EEG) electrode placement allows it to preferentially record over a cortical surface area. What is the approximate area covered by an EEG electrode?

    A $2 \, cm^2$
    B $4 \, cm^2$
    C $6 \, cm^2$
    D $8 \, cm^2$
    E $10 \, cm^2$

14. Which of the following statements about the sinusoidal waveform EEG is correct?

    A   Both extracellular and intracellular components are recorded on the EEG
    B   The waveform generated by direct excitatory and inhibitory interaction of neighbouring cortical cell columns
    C   The waveform is an indirect consequence of the additive effect of groups of cortical pyramidal neurons
    D   Polymorphic activity is usually sinusoidal
    E   There is variations in both the strength and the density of the current loops

NEUROSCIENCES: NEUROENDOCRINOLOGY

15. Which of the following describes cortisol accurately?

    A   Acts via dopamine receptors
    B   Elevated serum concentration in the morning
    C   Negative feedback on hypothalamus
    D   Positive feedback on pituitary
    E   Released from adrenal medulla

NEUROSCIENCES: NEUROCHEMISTRY

16. Which of the following is a monoamine neurotransmitter?

    A   Acetylcholine
    B   Growth hormone-releasing hormone
    C   Glycine
    D   Glutamate
    E   Neurotensin

17. Which of the following is the main effector of dopaminergic receptors?

    A D_1 – increase adenylyl cyclase
    B D_1 – decrease adenylyl cyclase
    C D_2 – increase adenylyl cyclase
    D D_3 – increase adenylyl cyclase
    E D_4 – increase adenylyl cyclase

18. Which of the following peptide secretions from neurons is released directly into the blood?

   A   Neurohormone
   B   Neuromediator
   C   Neuromodulator
   D   Neurotransmitter
   E   Neurotrophin

19. Which of the following is consistent with N-methyl-D-aspartate receptors?

   A   Excitatory amino acid neurotransmitter
   B   Binding site for γ-aminobutyric acid
   C   Hyperfunction associated with schizophrenia
   D   Metabotrophic receptor
   E   Type of glycine receptor

NEUROSCIENCES: NEUROIMAGING

20. A 67-year-old man underwent MRI recently. The scan showed focal atrophy of the caudate nucleus. What is the most likely diagnosis?

   A   Huntington's disease
   B   Hallervorden–Spatz disease
   C   Substance abuse including alcohol
   D   Long-term alcohol abuse
   E   Parkinson's disease

21. In which of the following conditions will MRI investigation show evidence of plaques in well over 90% of cases?

   A   Beçhet's disease
   B   Leukodystrophies
   C   Multiple sclerosis
   D   Normal ageing
   E   Sarcoidosis

22. Which of the following imaging modalities involves the BOLD technique?

   A   CT
   B   Functional MRI (fMRI)
   C   MRI
   D   Positron emission tomography (PET)
   E   Single photon emission computed tomography (SPECT)

23. Which of the following is used in clinical practice to measure glutamate, urea and ammonia?

   A ^{13}C
   B ^{14}N
   C ^{23}Na
   D ^{17}O
   E ^{31}P

PSYCHOPHARMACOLOGY: PHARMACOKINETICS

24. What is the mechanism of action of lofexidine?

    A α_2-Receptor agonist
    B α_2-Receptor antagonist
    C α_2-Receptor inverse agonist
    D   Monoamine reuptake inhibitor
    E   Serotonin reuptake inhibition

25. Which of the following drugs is a partial μ agonist?

    A   Buprenorphine
    B   Bupropion
    C   Buspirone
    D   Busulphan
    E   Butyrophenone

26. Which of the following statements applies to the pharmacokinetic properties of most psychotropic drugs?

    A   Most of them are affected by second-pass metabolism
    B   Most of them are minimally bound to proteins in the plasma
    C   They are poorly absorbed from the gut
    D   They are poorly ionised at a physiological pH
    E   They pass easily from plasma to the brain because they are hydrophilic

27. Which of the following statements about the effects of ageing on pharmacokinetics is correct?

    A   The receptor sensitivity is not affected
    B   The unbound proportion of albumin-bound drugs decreases
    C   The rate of absorption is increased
    D   The total amount of drug absorbed is reduced
    E   The volume of distribution increases for lipid-soluble drugs

28. Which of the following antipsychotics is not a substrate for cytochrome P450CYP450-2D6?

    A   Aripiprazole
    B   Clozapine
    C   Olanzapine
    D   Paliperidone
    E   Risperidone

29. Carbamazepine is not available as an intravenous injection. What is the most likely reason?

    A   It can cause severe allergic reaction
    B   It has a short half-life
    C   It is highly insoluble in water
    D   It is highly toxic as an intravenous preparation
    E   It rapidly distributes into all the tissues

30. A 32-year-old man had epilepsy. He was treated with carbamazepine 200 mg twice a day. His last serum carbamazepine levels were within normal limits. He was brought to the emergency department after a seizure and his carbamazepine levels were noticed to be low. He had been taking medication regularly, did not use illicit drugs or alcohol and was not on any other medication. What is the most likely explanation?

    A   Carbamazepine could be absorbed less in the intestine
    B   Carbamazepine induces its own metabolism
    C   Carbamazepine is highly water soluble
    D   Renal excretion of carbamazepine is increased
    E   There is no reason for his blood levels to be low

PSYCHOPHARMACOLOGY: PHARMACODYNAMICS

31. Which of the following explains varenicline's mechanism of action?

    A   Antagonist on serotonergic receptors
    B   Blocks dopamine receptors
    C   Inverse agonist on acetylcholine receptors
    D   Partial agonist on acetylcholine receptors
    E   Stimulating release of glutamate

32. Which of the following sets of benzodiazepines is correctly arranged in decreasing order of potency?

    A   Alprazolam, clonazepam, lorazepam, diazepam, midazolam
    B   Alprazolam, clonazepam, lorazepam, midazolam, diazepam
    C   Alprazolam, clonazepam, midazolam, lorazepam, diazepam
    D   Alprazolam, lorazepam, clonazepam, midazolam, diazepam
    E   Clonazepam, alprazolam, lorazepam, midazolam, diazepam

33. Which of the following is the most potent inhibitor of CYP450-2D6?

    A   Bupropion
    B   Duloxetine
    C   Fluvoxamine
    D   Reboxetine
    E   Sertraline

34. Which of the following statements explains the mechanism of action of sildenafil?

    A   By inducing the enzyme phosphodiesterase V, it raises the levels of cyclic guanosine monophosphate (cGMP)
    B   By inducing the enzyme phosphodiesterase V, it reduces the levels of cGMP
    C   By inhibiting the enzyme phosphodiesterase V, it raises the levels of cGMP
    D   By inhibiting the enzyme phosphodiesterase V, it reduces the levels of cGMP
    E   By inhibiting the enzyme phosphodiesterase V, it has no effect on the levels of cGMP

35. Which of the following explains the mechanism of action of zopiclone?

    A   Binding to γ-aminobutyric acid type A (GABA-A) and GABA-B receptors
    B   Non-selective binding to α-subunits of GABA-A receptors
    C   Selective binding to α_1-subunit of GABA-A receptors
    D   Selective binding to the γ subunit of GABA-C receptors
    E   Selective binding to the Z subunit of GABA-A receptors

36. A 34-year-old woman had depression. She was on fluoxetine 60 mg once a day. Her clinician reduced the dose to 40 mg a day and added mirtazapine 15 mg once a day. Next day, she developed fever, tachycardia, muscle twitches and confusion. Which of the following can explain this reaction?

   A   Idiosyncratic reaction
   B   Pharmacodynamic interaction
   C   Pharmacokinetic interaction
   D   Pharmacological agonism
   E   Pharmacological reaction

37. Which of the following statements about myristoylated alanine-rich C kinase substrate (MARCKS) is correct?

   A   MARCKS is a protein kinase substrate
   B   MARCKS is a substrate of carbamazepine
   C   MARCKS is implicated in the treatment of epilepsy
   D   MARCKS is implicated in the treatment of pain
   E   There is significant down-regulation of MARCKS with repeated use of carbamazepine

38. Which of the following anti-dementia drugs has the longest half-life?

   A   Donepezil
   B   Galantamine
   C   Memantine
   D   Rivastigmine
   E   Tacrine

PSYCHOPHARMACOLOGY: ADVERSE REACTIONS

39. Which of the following adverse effects of clozapine is independent of dose?

   A   Hypersalivation
   B   Hypotension
   C   Neutropenia
   D   Seizures
   E   Weight gain

40. Which of the following is a risk factor for QTc prolongation on an ECG and arrhythmia?

   A   Anorexia nervosa
   B   Hypermagnesaemia
   C   Male gender
   D   Right ventricular hypertrophy
   E   Tachycardia

41. A 43-year-old man with chronic schizophrenia is being treated with depot antipsychotic injections. He is seen in the outpatient clinic because he has had motor side effects. Which of the following is the most appropriate scale for a baseline assessment and subsequent follow-up?

   A   Barnes' akathisia rating scale
   B   Brief psychiatric rating scale
   C   Bush–Francis scale
   D   Simpson-Angus scale
   E   Unified Parkinson's disease rating scale

PSYCHOPHARMACOLOGY: THEORIES OF ACTION

42. Which of the following is the most appropriate drug to treat poststroke depression?

    A   Agomelatine
    B   Lofepramine
    C   Mianserin
    D   Mirtazapine
    E   Venlafaxine

43. Which of the following drugs is currently licensed in the UK for treatment of generalised anxiety disorder?

    A   Gabapentin
    B   Lamotrigine
    C   Pregabalin
    D   Tiagabin
    E   Vigabatrin

44. A 32-year-old woman with a past history of three manic episodes and one inpatient admission is stabilised on haloperidol and lithium. The last episode occurred 2 years ago. She has recently discovered that she is 6 weeks pregnant. What is the best course of action?

    A   Continue both the drugs without any change
    B   Continue haloperidol and lithium in reduced dosages
    C   Stop both the drugs and monitor patient closely
    D   Stop lithium and continue haloperidol
    E   Stop lithium and switch haloperidol to chlorpromazine

45. Who established that clozapine is effective in treating treatment-resistant schizophrenia?

    A   John Cade
    B   John Kane
    C   Max Fink
    D   Nancy Andreasen
    E   Pierre Deniker

PSYCHOPHARMACOLOGY: DRUG DEPENDENCE

46. Which of the following statements about disulfiram is correct?

    A   It inhibits alcohol dehydrogenase
    B   It is a reversible inhibitor of the enzyme
    C   It should be used at least 12 hours after the last alcohol ingestion
    D   Its use with alcohol can cause hypotension
    E   Its use with alcohol can lead to decreased levels of acetaldehyde in the blood

47. A 44-year-old man was admitted for alcohol detoxification. He has alcoholic cirrhosis of the liver and his blood investigations showed that his liver enzymes were raised. Which of the following drugs is most appropriate for detoxification?

    A   Carbamazepine
    B   Chlordiazepoxide
    C   Clonazepam
    D   Diazepam
    E   Oxazepam

GENETICS: CELLULAR AND MOLECULAR GENETICS

48. In which of the following stages of mitosis does the division of cytoplasm start?

    A   Anaphase
    B   Interphase
    C   Metaphase
    D   Prophase
    E   Telophase

49. Which genetic material is most suitable for postmortem studies of gene expression?

    A   DNA
    B   Gene
    C   mRNA
    D   Protein
    E   tRNA

50. Which of the following studies is appropriate to answer the question: 'What are the relative contributions of genes and environment?'

    A   Association analysis
    B   Family study
    C   Heritability study
    D   Linkage analysis
    E   Twin adoption study

51. What is the production of new copies of RNA from DNA called?

    A   Modification
    B   Replication
    C   Termination
    D   Transcription
    E   Translation

52. Which of the following statements about heritability in psychiatric genetics is correct?

    A   It is measured by the disconcordance rate among twin pairs
    B   It is a ratio of genetic variance to phenotypic variance
    C   It is a ratio of phenotypic variance to genetic variance
    D   It is the proportion of proband twins who have an affected co-twin
    E   It is the proportion of twin pairs when both of them are affected with the disorder

53. In the example, 'two relatives from same family sharing a common disorder have two alleles in common; one is at LOCI-1 and the other at LOC-2. Co-inheritance of these two alleles along with the disorder in the family tree suggests that some unobserved risk gene for the disorder is present near the loci'. What principle is applied in this case?

    A   Functional analysis
    B   Gene-dosage effect
    C   Genomic rearrangement
    D   Linkage analysis
    E   Linkage disequilibrium

54. Which of the following methods is used to determine whether a particular gene variant directly affects the risk for the disorder?

    A   Categorical gene analysis
    B   Genetic association analysis

    C   Genetic recombination analysis
    D   Genetic expressive analysis
    E   Genetic linkage analysis

55. Which of the following is correct if very tight linkage occurs between genetic markers in a haplotype?

    A   Logarithm of odd score will be 3 or 3+
    B   Markers will not undergo recombination and will be inherited together
    C   Markers will not undergo recombination and will not be inherited separately
    D   Markers will undergo recombination and will be inherited together
    E   Markers will undergo recombination and will not be inherited separately

56. What is the main difference between association studies and linkage studies?

    A   For association studies, the DNA marker has to be in the disease gene itself
    B   For linkage studies, the DNA marker has to be very tightly linked to the disease gene
    C   Linkage analysis has demonstrated strong links between the human leukocyte antigen system and several diseases
    D   Mutation analysis of polymorphisms is done by linkage analysis
    E   Association analysis can be used to 'scan the genome'

57. Which of the following statements about gene expression is correct?

    A   Genetic information flows from RNA to DNA to polypeptides
    B   Most genes encode peptides and are transcribed by RNA polymerase 2
    C   RNA splicing, capping and polyadenylation are pretranscriptional
    D   Tryptophan is specified by several codons
    E   Usual termination codon is AUG

GENETICS: BEHAVIOURAL GENETICS

58. What is the commonest cause of inherited learning disability?

    A   Down's syndrome
    B   Fragile X syndrome
    C   Phenylketonuria
    D   Trisomy X
    E   Tuberous sclerosis

59. Which of the following perturbations is most convincingly linked with aggregates in families in panic disorder of adults?

    A   Heart rate perturbations
    B   Respiratory perturbations
    C   Salivary fluid secretion perturbations
    D   Sweating rate perturbations
    E   Temperature regulation perturbations

60. In a third of children with autism, there is an increased peripheral level of a neurotransmitter. Which of the following neurotransmitters is implicated?

    A   Catecholamine
    B   Dopamine
    C γ-Aminobutyric acid
    D   Glutamate
    E   Serotonin

61. What is the percentage ratio genetic liability: depression by direct effect or indirect effect respectively?

    A   20:80
    B   40:60
    C   50:50
    D   60:40
    E   80:20

62. The concordance rate of bulimia nervosa in dizygotic twins is 30%. What is the likely concordance rate in monozygotic twins?

    A   15%
    B   35%
    C   45%
    D   50%
    E   55%

63. Which of the following terms describes the probability of manifestation of a disorder given a particular genotype?

    A   Ascertainment
    B   Expression
    C   Gamete imprinting
    D   Gamete penetrance
    E   Penetrance

GENETICS: ENDOPHENOTYPES

64. Which of the following personality traits is an endophenotype for suicide behaviour?

    A   Borderline – hysterical continuum
    B   Impulsive – assertiveness continuum
    C   Neuroticism
    D   Paranoid – schizoid continuum
    E   Schizoid – schizotypal continuum

65. Which of the following is the neurochemical endophenotype in suicidal behaviour?

    A   Cerebrospinal fluid 5-hydroxyindoleacetic acid A (5-HIAA) levels
    B   Serum 5-HIAA levels
    C   Serum cortisol levels
    D   Urinary vanillylmandelic acid levels
    E   Urinary 5-HIAA levels

66. Which of the following electroencephalogram (EEG) changes have been used as an endophenotype in linkage studies for alcohol dependence?

    A   Frontal δ activity
    B   K-complexes
    C   Low-voltage α activity
    D   Occipital Ω activity
    E   Spindle activity

GENETICS: GENETIC EPIDEMIOLOGY

67. Which of the following factors about the family history of alcoholism is correct?

A   Behavioural disturbances in childhood are associated with higher rates of alcoholism
B   Children of alcoholics are less likely to be exposed to high-risk environments
C   Female alcoholics with a family history of alcoholism have poorer outcomes
D   Late onset of alcoholism is associated with increased rates of alcoholism in the family
E   The rates of familial alcoholism are independent of socioeconomic status

68. Which of the following statements is one of the results of the Irish affected sibling pair study?

A   Alcohol dependence is environmentally mediated
B   Chromosomal variations in chromosome 14 are strongly related to alcoholism
C   Chromosomal variations in chromosome 3 are strongly related to alcoholism
D   Chromosomal variations in chromosome 4 are strongly related to alcoholism
E   Chromosomal variations in chromosome 21 are strongly related to alcoholism

69. In which of the following conditions is the effect of genetic predisposition strongest?

A   Anxiety disorders
B   Autism
C   Bipolar affective disorder
D   Eating disorder
E   Schizophrenia

70. Which of the following transcription factors is implicated in anxiety, alcohol abuse and substance dependence?

A   C-fos
B   C-Jun
C   CREB
D   FRA1
E   TATA motif

GENETICS: GENE–ENVIRONMENT INTERACTION

71. Which of the following statements about cannabis-induced psychosis is correct?

A   Cannabis misuse causing psychosis is an intoxication phenomenon
B   Cannabis misuse causing psychosis is reversible in all individuals
C   If a boy misuses cannabis from 11 years of age and stops in a year, the chances of developing psychosis are the same as in the general population
D   Individuals with the COMT (catechol-*O*-methyl transferase) gene *met/met* allele are at high risk of developing cannabis-induced psychosis
E   Individuals with the COMT gene *val/val* allele are at high risk of developing cannabis-induced psychosis

72. What does the term 'envirome' mean?

A   Internal as well as external environment of the individual
B   The environmental factors that predispose as well trigger psychiatric disorders
C   The immediate environment of an individual in which he or she lives
D   The internal environment of the individual that leads to a psychiatric disorder
E   The work and household environment of an individual that are stressful and lead to a psychiatric disorder

73. Abnormalities of chromosomes can lead to a psychosis that is similar to schizophrenia. Which of the following chromosomes is implicated in psychosis?

   A   Chromosome 16
   B   Chromosome 22
   C   Chromosome 4
   D   Chromosome 8
   E   Chromosome X

74. What does the term 'ontogenic niche' mean?

   A   The ecological and social settings that an individual shares with parents
   B   The ecological and social settings that an individual shares with peers
   C   The ecological environment in which a person lives that modifies the genes
   D   The internal environment of an individual that modifies the genes
   E   The social environment in which a person lives that modifies the genes

75. You conducted a family study of patients with recurrent depressive disorder. Your findings showed that there was an increased risk of developing depression in parents' siblings and offsprings as probands, whereas second- and third-degree relatives do not have the increased risk. What does this mean?

   A   Environmental factors play a more important role in the development of depression than genetic factors
   B   Genetic factors play a more important role in the development of depression than environment
   C   There is no role for environmental factors in the development of depression
   D   There is no role for genetic factors in the development of depression
   E   This finding does not give any conclusive evidence as to whether genetic or environmental factors play a major role in the development of depression

EPIDEMIOLOGY: SURVEYS ACROSS THE LIFESPAN

76. What is the 12-month prevalence of mental disorders in Europe?

   A   1 in 4
   B   1 in 6
   C   1 in 10
   D   1 in 20
   E   1 in 100

77. According to a 10-year follow-up study of patients with borderline personality disorder, what is the median time to remission of the abandonment symptom?

   A   0–2 years
   B   2–4 years
   C   4–6 years
   D   6–8 years
   E   8–10 years

78. What is the reported prevalence of late-onset paraphrenia among elderly people in the community?

   A   <1%
   B   1–5%
   C   5–10%
   D   10–15%
   E   >15%

79. What is the prevalence of late-onset paraphrenia in elderly people in a psychiatric hospital population?

A   5%
B   10%
C   25%
D   20%
E   25%

80. If the prevalence of dementia is to be reduced by 50%, by how many years should the onset of dementia need to be delayed?

A   2 years
B   5 years
C   7 years
D   10 years
E   15 years

81. Elimination of depression from the elderly population can lead to a reduction in the number of new cases over a period of 7 years. What is the mean reduction expected?

A   5%
B   7%
C   10%
D   12%
E   15%

82. With regard to problem behaviour in patients with learning disability, which of the following is correct?

A   Common in females
B   Mainly one type of problem behaviour found
C   Prevalence of 10–15%
D   Prevalent in 30- to 45-year age group
E   Tendency to be short-lived

83. Which of the following statements about alcohol-related dementia is correct?

A   Early onset is associated with a poor prognosis
B   It accounts for 15% of the dementia population
C   It occurs more in areas of high socioeconomic status
D   It presents most commonly at the age of 40–50 years
E   The prevalence of Wernicke's aphasia/Korsakoff's syndrome is on the decrease

84. Which one of the following is not a predictor of course and outcome in schizophrenia?

A   Characteristics of the onset of the illness
B   Features of initial clinical state and treatment response
C   First rank symptoms at the baseline
D   History of past psychotic episodes and treatment
E   Premorbid personality and functioning

85. Which of the following statements about a cross-sectional study is correct?

A   It is bias free
B   It can explore multiple outcomes and exposures
C   It is hard to design
D   It is suitable for rare conditions
E   It takes a long time to complete

86. Which of the following statements is a characteristic feature of a qualitative study?

    A   It is based on experiments
    B   It is based on a survey
    C   It is deductive
    D   It is useful to generate a hypothesis
    E   The sampling method used is statistical

87. The suicide rate has increased worldwide in the last 45 years. Which of the following reflects the increased rate?

    A   20%
    B   30%
    C   40%
    D   50%
    E   60%

88. In which age group was the suicide rate highest by sex and age in the UK from 2000 to 2009?

    A   15–44 years: males
    B   15–44 years: females
    C   45–74 years: females
    D   45–74 years: males
    E   75+ years: males/females

EPIDEMIOLOGY: MEASURES

89. What is the cross-sectional observation of the number of individuals with a disease in a specified population called?

    A   Incidence
    B   Life-time prevalence
    C   Prevalence
    D   Period prevalence
    E   Point prevalence

90. A disease under study has a high prevalence. What is the most likely possibility?

    A   High incidence, short duration of disease
    B   High incidence, long duration of disease
    C   Low incidence, short duration of disease
    D   Low incidence, long duration of disease
    E   Low incidence due to rare disease

91. What is the number of new cases of a disease over a period of time out of the total population at risk called?

    A   Cumulative incidence
    B   Incidence rate
    C   Incidence density
    D   Period prevalence
    E   Point prevalence

92. What does comparing observed deaths to expected deaths signify?

    A   Crude mortality rate
    B   Odds ratio

C   Relative risk
D   Specific mortality rate
E   Standardised mortality ratio

93. Which of the following rating scales is a self-rating scale to measure symptom severity and change in a mental illness?

A   Beck's depression inventory
B   Brief psychiatric rating scale
C   Clinical global improvement scale
D   Hamilton's rating scale for depression
E   Yale–Brown obsessive–compulsive scale (Y-BOCS)

94. Which of the following statements about the Y-BOCS is correct?

A   It also measures anxiety
B   It is a diagnostic tool
C   It is useful to assess obsessions
D   It is useful to monitor the response to treatment
E   It is used only in research settings

95. What is the tendency of a rater to overestimate a patient's response based on prior assumptions called?

A   Ceiling effect
B   Central limit theorem
C   Ecological fallacy
D   Halo effect
E   Hawthorne effect

96. What is the denominator in maternal mortality rate?

A   1000 live births
B   10,000 live births
C   100,000 live births
D   All live births + still births
E   All live births + still births + perinatal deaths

ADVANCED PSYCHOLOGICAL PROCESSES AND TREATMENTS: NEUROPSYCHOLOGY

97. Which of the following statements about memory is correct?

A   Encoding is related to concepts of memory storage
B   Long-term memory is also known as working memory
C   Long-term memory has unlimited capacity
D   Transfer of memory to long-term memory begins 30 minutes after information enters short-term memory
E   Unless rehearsed, storage in short-term memory is limited to 30 seconds

98. Which of the following statements about neurocognition in schizophrenia is correct?

A   Attention-processing speed is impaired more than the executive function domain
B   Deterioration in IQ is more rapid after the first episode of schizophrenia than the subsequent episodes
C   Deficits in motor skills are more pronounced than in the verbal memory domain

    D   Illness chronicity accounts for most cognitive impairments in schizophrenia
    E   Neurocognitive impairments usually begin after the first episode of schizophrenia

ADVANCED PSYCHOLOGICAL PROCESSES AND TREATMENTS: PERSONALITY AND PERSONALITY DISORDER

99. Which of the following statements about assessing the personality of an individual is correct?

    A   This involves giving short-term acquaintances questionnaires
    B   The Minnesota multiphasic personality inventory is a poorly researched inventory
    C   The best method is by observation made during an episode of illness
    D   The trait approach is considered to be the most reliable method of assessment
    E   The trait approach to personality assessment is the basis for the ICD-10 classification

100. A mother of a 7-year-old boy kept giving him laxatives in his food covertly and frequently took him to the hospital and insisted on his admission. Which of the following statements about this situation is correct?

    A   It is considered child maltreatment, according to definitions used by the government in England and Wales
    B   Personality disorder is commonly observed among the perpetrators
    C   The child won't be harmed because he is being cared for in hospital
    D   This is best considered a form of parental psychopathology
    E   This is exploitation of a vulnerable and defenceless child

ADVANCED PSYCHOLOGICAL PROCESSES AND TREATMENTS: DEVELOPMENTAL PSYCHOPATHOLOGY INCLUDING TEMPERAMENT

101. According to current evidence, which of the following statements about the development of puberty compared with previous generations is correct?

    A   Average age of menarche has reduced to below 11 years
    B   One in four girls reaches puberty before the age of 8 years
    C   One in ten 8-year-old boys has pubic hair
    D   Puberty lasts longer than in previous generations
    E   There is no change in the age of maturation of boys

102. According to the New York longitudinal study, what percentage of the cohort was identified as having an easy temperament?

    A   10%
    B   15%
    C   20%
    D   35%
    E   40%

103. Which of the following statements about authoritarian parenting is correct?

    A   Children are popular and sociable
    B   Children have poor impulse control

    C   Non-negotiable parents who are strict
    D   Parents are willing to discuss with children
    E   Parents do not set limits

104. A girl was placed in a day care at the age of 6 months when her mother returned to part-time work of 24 hours a week. According to Bowlby, what is the most likely effect on her around her first birthday?

    A   Attachment is unaffected
    B   Child experiences maternal deprivation
    C   Object permanence does not develop
    D   Privation is not possible
    E   Child's response in strange situation test shows a disorganised attachment

105. The adult attachment interview is a tool used in research. Which of the following statements is correct about this tool?

    A   Five possible attachment styles can be identified
    B   It identifies attachment relationships during adulthood
    C   It is a semi-structured interview
    D   Studies use it in the context of intergenerational transfer of attachment patterns
    E   It is used mainly to identify the individual who might have been sexually abused as a child

106. Which of the following statements about object relations theory is correct?

    A   It includes the paranoid–depressive positions
    B   Only external object relations can be achieved
    C   The work was lead primarily by Sigmund Freud
    D   The paranoid–depressive positions are never fully resolved in adult life
    E   It uses defence mechanisms such as sexualisation and idealisation

107. Who described the 'good-enough mother'?

    A   Bowlby
    B   Freud
    C   Jung
    D   Klein
    E   Winnicott

ADVANCED PSYCHOLOGICAL PROCESSES AND TREATMENTS: THERAPY MODELS, METHODS, PROCESSES AND OUTCOMES

108. Which of the following statements about condensation in dream analysis is correct?

    A   Dream content substitutes the target of one's feelings onto another person or object
    B   It is also called dramatisation
    C   It makes sense of the manifest content
    D   It refers to what we dream about and are aware of on waking
    E   More than one dream idea is combined into a single mental image

109. Which of the following statements is about neurotic symptoms in psychoanalysis?

    A   They are considered by Freud to be the 'secret road to the unconscious'
    B   Dreams have different meanings from neurotic symptoms

C   The symptoms may symbolise the wish with which they are linked
D   The symptoms are often 'mental'
E   The underlying cause is rarely 'physical'

110. Which of the following describes snags in cognitive–analytical therapy?

A   Accurate description of autonomic procedures
B   Appropriate roles or goals abandoned because they are perceived as forbidden or dangerous.
C   Available action or possible roles limited to polarised alternatives
D   Negative assumptions which generate acts that reinforce the assumptions
E   Patient helped to recognise recurrences of unrevised patterns

111. A 32-year-old man was reprimanded by his boss, although he did not react at the time. When he went home, he shouted at his wife and slapped her after a minor argument. What is the likely defence mechanism?

A   Denial
B   Displacement
C   Humour
D   Reaction formation
E   Sublimation

112. According to jungian psychoanalysis, which of the following statements refers to consciousness?

A   It has four basic functions
B   It is accessible through recall
C   It includes archetypes
D   It is made up of the individual's unique experiences involving repression
E   It includes the mind's inherited characteristics that influence the reactions

113. In Yalom's universal therapeutic factors, catharsis refers to which of the following?

A   Expression of affect in a supportive environment
B   Filled with therapeutic optimism by seeing others improve
C   Improving one's self-esteem by helping another
D   Model helpful behaviours of other members
E   Recognition of common experiences and that it reflects experiences in wider society

114. Which of the following statements best describes the technique of paradoxical injunction used in systemic family therapy?

A   Different positions are assigned to parts of the family structure
B   Members of the family are 'prescribed' their symptom which can paradoxically lead to an alteration
C   Practical solutions are developed between family members
D   Tasks are assigned to family members to complete between sessions, which involve a change in their actions to see how it affects the system
E   Thought is given to how to live with symptoms if they cannot be altered

115. Which of the following therapies is the treatment of choice for anorexia nervosa in adolescents?

A   Exposure response and reciprocal inhibition
B   Eye-movement desensitisation and reprocessing
C   Psychodynamic psychotherapy
D   Systemic desensitisation
E   Systemic family therapy

116. A 20-year-old woman recently diagnosed with moderate depression would prefer a psychological therapy rather than taking medication. Which of the following therapies should be recommended?

A   Brief solution-focused therapy
B   Cognitive–behavioural therapy (CBT)
C   Psychodynamic interpersonal therapy
D   Supportive counselling
E   Systemic family therapy

117. A 26-year-old school teacher felt that she was responsible for every child in her class passing the examination, otherwise her colleagues would view her as a failure. Which of the following cognitive errors does she have?

A   Assuming temporal causality
B   Catastrophising
C   Excessive responsibility
D   Dichotomous thinking
E   Over-generalising

118. Which of the following statements about dialectical behavioural therapy is correct?

A   It can extend for a maximum of 6 months
B   It was developed by Linehan
C   It involves exploring childhood adversity with a therapist through free association
D   It involves only group work
E   The therapy is intensive with group and individual work

119. Which of the following is one of the stages of eye-movement desensitisation and reprocessing?

A   Awareness
B   Competing response
C   Contingency management
D   Habit reversal training
E   Target assessment

ADVANCED PSYCHOLOGICAL PROCESSES AND TREATMENTS: TREATMENT ADHERENCE

120. Which of the following statements about the National Institute for Health and Care Excellence's guideline for a stepped care approach to generalised anxiety disorder is correct?

A   Step 2 – identification and assessment
B   Step 3 – low-intensity psychological interventions
C   Step 3 – day hospital or inpatient care can be considered
D   Step 4 – considered if there is high risk of self-harm
E   Step 5 – CBT or drug treatment can be initiated

121. Which of the following statements about psychological treatments for people with an antisocial personality disorder (ASPD) is correct?

A   Most of the psychological interventions delivered in the criminal justice system are largely based on concepts of conditioning
B   Psychological interventions for almost all of the components of ASPD are well developed

    C   Roughly half of all interventions delivered in the criminal justice system are aimed at reducing offending behaviour

    D   There has been significant formal development of psychological interventions for ASPD

    E   There is a good research base for psychological management for comorbid disorders seen in ASPD

122. Which of the following statements about combined CBT and antidepressants is correct?

    A   After ending treatment, relapse rates of depression are similar in those treated with either CBT or antidepressants

    B   CBT is as effective as antidepressant medication in depressed inpatients

    C   Drug treatments have a higher relapse rate than CBT on discontinuation in generalised anxiety disorder

    D   The combination of CBT and antidepressant medication may be as effective as either alone in severe depression

    E   The combination of CBT and medication in mild-to-moderate depression is more effective than either alone

123. Which of the following treatments is harmful in post-traumatic stress disorder?

    A   Counselling
    B   Debriefing
    C   Drug treatment
    D   Trauma-focused CBT
    E   Eye-movement desensitisation and reprocessing

124. A 44-year-old woman complained of intense and irrational fears about eating in front of other people. Her therapist arranged a session at which she consumed a meal in front of four strangers. During the session, they looked at her but did not talk to her. However, she occasionally observed them whispering to each other. What type of therapy has been described?

    A   Assertiveness training
    B   Flooding
    C   Habit reversal
    D   Relaxation therapy
    E   Systemic desensitisation

125. Which of the following is an inclusion criterion for group therapy?

    A   Inability to tolerate group setting
    B   Motivation to change
    C   Problem areas incompatible with group goals
    D   Severe incompatibility with one or more group members
    E   Tendency to assume deviant role

126. A 20-year-old female college student repeatedly self-harmed, expressed feelings of being miserable, lonely and abandoned by family and friends. She found it difficult to maintain romantic relationships. Which of the following is the most appropriate psychological therapy for treatment?

    A   CBT
    B   Counselling
    C   Dialectical behavioural therapy
    D   Systemic desensitisation
    E   Systemic family therapy

ADVANCED PSYCHOLOGICAL PROCESSES AND TREATMENTS: PSYCHOSOCIAL INFLUENCES

127. Which of the following statements is consistent with emotional deprivation in children?

A   A child will show either clinging or detachment after short-term deprivation
B   After long-term deprivation children become self-sufficient through detachment
C   Long-term deprivation includes a child going to stay with grandparents, while the mother is on holiday
D   Short-term deprivation includes separation after a divorce
E   There are no long-term effects of short-term deprivation in children

128. Which of the following is a risk factor related to the parent/environment for child abuse?

A   Being abused as a child
B   Good socioeconomic status and high-powered job of parents
C   High self-esteem in parents
D   Older age of parents
E   Small family size

129. Which of the following statements about couples and divorce in the UK is correct?

A   About 60% of couples cohabit before they marry
B   After divorce, men have a lower rate of remarriage than women
C   Couples who cohabit before marriage are unlikely to divorce later
D   Divorce rates peak after 10–12 years of marriage
E   Divorce rates are highest in individuals in late 30s

130. Which of the following vulnerability factors in parents is considered in identifying children at risk of developing conduct problems?

A   All mothers are younger than 18 years
B   At least one of the parents is on social security benefits
C   At least one parent has a degree of contact with the criminal justice system
D   Parents have an education status below the GCSE level
E   Parents have other mental health problems

131. Which of the following statements about association between sexual abuse and psychiatric disorder is correct?

A   Girls are more prone to psychiatric disorders than boys after sexual abuse
B   A history of rape does not add any more to the risks of a psychiatric disorder if sexual abuse had already occurred
C   Patients are more prone to psychiatric disorders when they were abused before the age of 10 years compared with after the age of 15 years
D   There is enough evidence to show an association between sexual abuse and obsessive–compulsive disorder
E   There is a statistically significant association between sexual abuse and lifetime diagnosis of sleep disorders

Answers: MCQs

1. E Schwann cells

Neuroglial cells surround the neurons providing them with support and protection. They play a significant role in phagocytosis and myelin production. Neuroglial cells are of two main types known as microglia and macroglia. Microglia are specialised macrophages found in the central nervous system (CNS) whereas macroglia are found in both CNS and the peripheral nervous system (PNS). Schwann cell s, satellite cells and enteric glial cells are macroglia found in the PNS. Astrocytes, ependymal cells, oligodendrocytes and radial glial cells are macroglia found in the CNS. The most abundant type of macroglia in the PNS is the Schwann cells. However, overall, the most abundant type of macroglia is astrocytes.

2. E Oligodendroglioma

Intrinsic brain tumours include various grades of glioma, astrocytoma, oligodendroglioma, medulloblastoma, lymphoma and ependymoma. Oligodendroglioma is found in 10% of adults and 4% of children with primary brain tumour. The most common form of astrocytoma is gliobastoma multiforme. Extrinsic brain tumours include meningioma, neuroma, epidermoid tumour, glomus jugulare and chordoma.

3. B Cerebellum

Dentate nucleus is one of the four deep cerebellar nuclei that connect cerebellum to other regions of brain. It is phylogenetically the most recent and lateral nuclei. It is located in deep white matter. Other three deep cerebellar nuclei are called fastigial, globose and emboliform nuclei. The largest deep cerebellar nucleus is dentate nucleus and the smallest is an interposed nucleus which is a combined globose and emboliform nucleus.

4. A 5, 7

Astereognosia is associated with a lesion in the somatosensory association cortex that is located in Brodmann's areas 5 and 7. Loss of saccadic eye movement and impaired visual search is linked to lesions in the frontal eye fields (Brodmann's area 8) and dorsolateral prefrontal cortex (Brodmann's area 9). Impulsive behaviour and perseveration can be seen as a result of lesions in the dorsolateral prefrontal cortex (Brodmann's area 9) and anterior prefrontal cortex (Brodmann's area 10). Visual object agnosia is related to lesions in the secondary visual cortex (Brodmann's area 18), associative visual cortex (Brodmann's area 19) and inferior temporal gyrus (Brodmann's area 20). Auditory agnosia can occur as a result of lesions in the superior temporal gyrus (Brodmann's area 22) and primary auditory cortex (Brodmann's area 42).

5. C Alexia and agraphia

The lesion in area 6 is associated with agraphia without alexia and those in areas 7 and 40 are associated with Gerstmann's syndrome. Lesions 18 and 19 can cause alexia without agraphia. However, lesions 39 and 40, and the frontal lobe lesion can cause acalculia. The lesion in area 22 gives rise to Wernicke's aphasia.

6. C Parahippocampal gyrus is significantly smaller

Neuroimaging studies have found that parahippocampal gyrus is smaller in patients with schizophrenia compared with controls. Other structural changes noticed in schizophrenia include reduction in the brain mass, temporal lobe, cerebral volumes and overall brain length. There is ventricular enlargement, particularly involving the temporal horn. There is no significant difference in the hippocampal area.

7. C Perforation of the septum pellucidum

Punch-drunk syndrome, also known as boxer's dementia or dementia pugilistica, occurs in professional boxers who are subjected to repeated blows, resulting in concussions. It is a neurodegenerative disease in which individuals present with symptoms suggestive of dementia, parkinsonism, memory loss, and gait and speech problems. On macroscopic examination of the postmortem brain there is evidence of perforation of the septum pellucidum, cerebral atrophy, ventricular enlargement, thinning of the corpus callosum, brain tissue scarring and hydrocephalus. On microscopic examination there is evidence of neuronal loss, collections of senile plaques and neurofibrillary tangles.

8. E Temporal lobe

Macroscopic changes in Alzheimer's disease include global brain atrophy, ventricular brain enlargement and widening of the sulci. In this disease, atrophy is most significant in the frontal and temporal lobes of the brain. In Pick's disease, histopathological changes are noticed in cerebral cortex, basal ganglia, locus ceruleus and substantia nigra.

9. B Knife blade gyri

Pick's disease is a rare neurodegenerative disorder. In this disorder there is asymmetrical atrophy of the frontal and temporal lobes with sparing of the occipital and parietal lobes. The cerebral atrophy is so severe that some of the gyri are extremely thin, which is also known as knife blade gyri. In this disease, ventricles are enlarged. In Alzheimer's disease, there is global brain atrophy and sulcal widening.

10. A Generalised cerebral atrophy

Creutzfeldt–Jakob disease (CJD) is a fatal degenerative brain disease.

CJD is transmitted by infection with a prion, which is a protein in misfolded form. There are several types of CJD such as sporadic, variant, familial and iatrogenic types. In CJD there is selective cerebellar atrophy, generalised cerebral atrophy and ventricular enlargement. On histopathological examination there is a spongiform appearance to the brain tissue due to death of nerve cells. Neurofibrillary tangles, neuritic plaques and neuronal loss are histological changes found in dementia caused by Lewy bodies.

11. A Combined growth hormone-releasing hormone and somatostatins

Growth hormone is secreted by somatotrophic cells which are located within the anterior pituitary gland. It is under the stimulatory effect of growth hormone-releasing factor (GHRH or somatocrinin) and the inhibitory effect of somatostatins, both of which are released from neurosecretory cells in the hypothalamus. There are a number of other factors such as diet, age, gender, physical activity and stress that influence secretion of growth hormone.

12. C Glutamate receptors

The ion channels are classified into families on the basis of genetic sequence, homology and possibly pore lining α-sub unit type. The main families are transmembrane agents (6 TM, 4/8 TM, 2 TM), inotropic glutamate receptors, nicotinic-related receptors, intracellular calcium ion channels and chloride ion channels. Glutamate receptor is a ligand-gated ion channel. The sodium, potassium and calcium channels are ion-gated channels.

13. C 6 cm^2

International 10–20 system is a recognised system that describes the electrode placement on the scalp in an electroencephalogram (EEG) investigation. In this system, the scalp is divided into a grid that helps in compensating for the different head size in different patients. Each electrode records approximately 6 cm^2 of the cortical area.

14. E Variation in both the strength and the density of the current loops

Waveforms on an EEG can be monomorphic, polymorphic, sinusoidal or transient. The variations in both strength and density of the current loops lead to development of the characteristic sinusoidal waveform. Monomorphic activity is most likely to be sinusoidal waves. The cortical pyramidal neurons are arranged in radial columns and are directed outward. The membrane potential of the columns fluctuate, as a result of which an electric 'dipole' is generated. This dipole results in an electrical field potential as current flows through both extracellular and intercellular space. The waveform is generated by reciprocal excitatory and inhibitory interaction of neighbouring cortical cell columns. The extracellular component of the current is recorded in the EEG.

15. C Negative feedback on hypothalamus

Cortisol has a negative feedback effect on the hypothalamus, hippocampus and pituitary gland. It is a glucocorticoid steroid hormone that is secreted by zona fasciculata found in the adrenal cortex. It acts via glucocorticoid receptor types I and II. It is secreted in response to exposure to stress. Cortisol levels vary with diurnal changes. It is raised in serum just after awakening and is low in the evenings.

16. A Acetylcholine

A monoamine neurotransmitter can be both a neurotransmitter and a neuromodulator. Aromatic amino acids such as phenylalanince, tryptophan, thyroid hormones and tyrosine produce monoamine neurotransmitters. Dopamine, noradrenaline, adrenaline, serotonin, acetylcholine and histamine are the monoamine receptors. GHRH, glycine and glutamate are the amino acid receptors. Endorphins, cholecystokinin, angiotensin II, neurotensin and corticotrophin-releasing hormone are peptide neurotransmitters.

17. A D$_1$ increase adenylyl cyclase

The dopamine receptors are coupled to G-proteins. The main effectors of dopamine receptors are D1 which increases adenylyl cyclase, D2 which decreases adenylyl cyclase, D3 which decreases adenylyl cyclase, D4 which decreases adenylyl cyclase and D5 which increases adenylyl cyclase.

18. A Neurohormone

A neurohormone is a peptide secretion from neuroendocrine cells. It is released directly into the blood and reaches the systemic circulation, e.g. corticotrophin-releasing hormone.

A neurotransmitter is a substance found in and released from a neuron, which thereby transmits an impulse from one neuron to another neuron, e.g. acetylcholine.

A neuromodulator is a substance that originates from a postsynaptic site and either potentiates or inhibits neuronal transmission, e.g. steroid hormones.

A neuromediator is a postsynaptic substance that results in postsynaptic response, e.g. second messenger such as cAMP.

A neurotrophin is a protein substance, again from a postsynaptic site, but it maintains a presynaptic neuronal structure and induces the survival, development and function of neurons, e.g. nerve growth factor.

19. A Excitatory amino acid neurotransmitter

N-Methyl-D-aspartate (NMDA) is a type of glutamate receptor, and an excitatory amino acid neurotransmitter. Although glutamate activates both ligand-gated ion channels (ionotropic) and G-protein coupled receptors (metabotropic), NMDA is exclusively ionotropic. It has binding sites for glycine and phencyclidine. It has been hypothesised that schizophrenia results from the hypofunction of NMDA.

20. A Huntington's disease

Focal atrophy of the caudate nucleus is often seen on CT or MRI in Huntington's disease. As the illness progresses cerebral atrophy is noticed on neuroimaging. In MRI the characteristic areas of low signal are seen due to abnormal deposition of iron in the basal nuclei in Huntington's disease and Hallervorden–Spatz disease. Alcohol and illicit drug use can give rise to specific atrophy of the cerebellum.

21. C Multiple sclerosis

Neuroimaging, mainly MRI, is helpful in diagnosis and follow-up of patients with multiple sclerosis. It is the commonest cause of demyelination in the CNS and involves the brain's white matter. MRI will show evidence of plaques in well over 90% of the cases, although the location varies because it can affect practically any part of the brain. It is usually difficult to demonstrate white matter disease using CT or MRI. The demonstration of small foci of increased signal (T2-weighted images) is possibly due to demyelination but it could be a non-specific finding seen in a vascular and inflammatory condition such as Behçet's disease or sarcoidosis. In the leukodystrophies, the symmetrical involvement of white matter is usually a characteristic feature.

22. B MRI

A technique that is dependent on the blood oxygenation level is used in functional MRI (fMRI) to detect images that are based on cerebral blood flow and regional activity. When an area of the brain is functionally active due to a task, there is an initial decrease in oxygenated haemoglobin and an increase in deoxygenated haemoglobin and carbon dioxide. After few seconds (2–6 seconds) of neuronal activity, there is an increase in cerebral blood flow to this area of brain, leading to an increase in local oxygenated haemoglobin concentration. It is this level of change in oxygenated haemoglobin that is detected by fMRI. It therefore detects the functionally active brain regions.

23. B ^{14}N

Magnetic resonance spectroscopy (MRS) is used to measure metabolic changes in conditions such as stroke, brain tumours, Alzheimer's dementia and other neurological illnesses. It can also be used to measure metabolic changes in muscle by detecting intramyocellular lipid. MRS involves the use of different nuclei, which in a magnetic field absorbs and emits electromagnetic radiation. ^{14}N is used in the measurement of glutamate, urea and ammonia. ^{13}C and ^{17}O are used in the analysis of metabolite turnover rate. ^{23}Na is used for the study of intracellular sodium metabolism. ^{31}P is used in the analysis of bioenergetics, identification of unusual metabolites and measurement of pH.

24. A α_2-Receptor agonist

Opioids inhibit noradrenaline release, and discontinuation of opioids causes a rebound release of noradrenaline. Lofexidine, an α_2-adrenoceptor agonist, acts by reducing the noradrenergic storm that follows discontinuation of opioids. Stimulation of α_2-autoreceptors inhibits noradrenergic release. Therefore, it is indicated in treating opioid withdrawal.

25. A Buprenorphine

Mu (μ) receptors are opioid receptors. Buprenorphine is a partial μ agonist opioid, used for analgesia and treatment of opioid dependence. Bupropion is an antidepressant that acts as a noradrenaline and dopamine reuptake inhibitor antidepressant. Buspirone is an anxiolytic that acts as a 5-hydroxytryptamine 1A partial agonist. Butyrophenone is a class of antipsychotic drugs that includes benperidol and haloperidol. Busulphan is a chemotherapy agent.

26. D They are poorly ionised at physiological pH

Ionisation of drugs is largely dependent on the pH of the solution. It affects the absorption, distribution and elimination of drugs in the body. Antipsychotics are not highly ionised at physiological pH. In general, most psychotropic drugs are easily absorbed from the gut and they pass from the plasma to the brain due to their lipophilic property. Most of them are metabolised in the liver and are affected by first-pass metabolism. They are largely bound to proteins in the plasma, but only plasma-free fractions are pharmacologically active.

27. E Volume of distribution increases for lipid-soluble drugs

Total body water and lean body mass decrease in old age, whereas total body fat increases. This leads to an increase in volume of distribution (V_d) for lipid-soluble drugs but a decreased Vd for water-soluble drugs. Receptor sensitivity may increase in old age, leading to increased effects of the drugs. Due to delayed gastric emptying and slow motility, absorption is usually slowed down but just as complete. The albumin level decreases so the proportion of free or unbound drug increases. Half-lives are usually prolonged.

28. D Paliperidone

This is metabolised by the cytochrome P450 CYP450-2D6 into its active metabolite, paliperidone. Therefore, paliperidone itself is not a substrate for this enzyme. All the other antipsychotics mentioned in the question are metabolised by this enzyme. Therefore, in theory, their dose should be reduced when a CYP450-2D6 inhibitor (e.g. fluoxetine, paroxetine, duloxetine) is administered concomitantly. In the case of risperidone, it increases the risk of extrapyramidal side effects. Paliperidone injection is indicated for maintenance in patients with schizophrenia who had previously responded to risperidone or paliperidone tablets.

29. C It is highly insoluble in water

Carbamazepine is poorly soluble in water and most other liquids. Hence, it has been difficult to develop an intravenous formulation. However, recently a University of Minnesota group has developed intravenous carbamazepine using cyclodextrins. A study published in 2009 suggested that the intravenous formulation was safe, although it will be long before it is available for use in patients. Carbamazepine dissolves rapidly into the tissues with 70–80% plasma bound. It has a half-life of 26 hours (18–54 hours) after the first dose.

30. B Carbamazepine induces its own metabolism

Carbamazepine is an enzyme inducer and can induce its own metabolism. This is called autoinduction. The half-life of carbamazepine after a single dose is 26 hours (18–54 hours). After repeated use it can be decreased to 5–26 hours.

31. D Partial agonist on acetylcholine receptors

Varenicline is a partial agonist of nicotine acetylcholine receptor. It is used in people who wish to stop smoking. By its partial agonist activity on the $\alpha_4\beta_2$-subtype of nicotine receptor, it helps in reducing the craving and withdrawal symptoms of smoking. Furthermore, it can reduce the positive effects of smoking, thereby helping a smoker to quit.

32. B Alprazolam, clonazepam, lorazepam, midazolam, diazepam

Table 1.1 describes the equivalent dose of commonly used benzodiazepines. The lower the equivalent dose, the higher the potency of the drug.

Table 1.1 Dose equivalents (DEs) of benzodiazepines	
Commonly used benzodiazepine drugs	**Dose equivalents (lower the DE, higher the potency)**
Alprazolam	0.25
Clonazepam	0.5
Lorazepam	1
Midazolam	0.25–1.7
Diazepam	5
Temazepam	5
Chlordiazepoxide	10
Oxazepam	15

33. B Duloxetine

CYP450-2D6 enzyme metabolises various antidepressants including tricyclic antidepressants (TCAs), duloxetine and selective serotonin reuptake inhibitors (SSRIs). It also converts venlafaxine into its active metabolite, desvenlafaxine. Paroxetine, duloxetine and fluoxetine are its potent inhibitors whereas other SSRIs, reboxetine and bupropion are among its weak inhibitors.

Concomitant administration of TCAs and SSRIs may require a dose reduction of TCAs. Concomitant administration of CYP450-2D6 inhibitors can also interfere with the analgesic effect of codeine.

34. C By inhibiting the enzyme phosphodiesterase V, it raises the levels of cGMP

Normally cyclic guanosine monophosphate (cGMP) causes smooth muscle relaxation, resulting in a physiological erection. The cGMP is broken down in the penis by phosphodiesterase-V enzyme. Sildenafil inhibits the enzyme, so helping the levels of cGMP to build up in the penis, leading to an erection. A desire to have sex is essential for sildenafil to work, meaning that it will not work during sleep.

35. B Non-selective binding to α-subunits of GABA-A receptors

There are three types of γ-aminobutyric acid (GABA) receptors: GABA-A, GABA-B and GABA-C. GABA-A receptors have different subtypes depending on the subunits: α (1–6), β (1–3), γ (1–3), δ, ε, π, Ω and ρ (1–3). Zopiclone, eszopiclone and benzodiazepines bind to $α_1$, $α_2$, $α_3$ and $α_5$ subunits of GABA-A receptors. Alpha-1 subtype is critical for sedation and is also linked to daytime sedation, anticonvulsant action and amnesia. Zaleplon and zolpidem are selective to the $α_1$-subtype and so have less risk of tolerance and dependence.

36. B Pharmacodynamic interaction

Pharmacodynamics is the study of the biochemical and physiological effects of the drug on the body. Pharmacodynamic interaction happens when drugs that have same or opposing action are given together. These drugs may alter the sensitivity or response of the body to the drugs. There are some reports of serotonin syndrome due to an interaction between mirtazapine and fluoxetine when co-administered.

37. A MARCKS is a protein kinase substrate

This is an abbreviation for myristoylated alanine-rich C kinase substrate (MARCKS) protein. Recent studies show that the mood-stabilising effect of mood stabilisers are attributed to the effect of medication on MARCKS. It has been noticed that with use of sodium valproate and lithium there is a significant down-regulation of MARCKS expression. Carbamazepine lacks this effect, indicating that the mechanism of mood stabilisation of carbamazepine is different to that of lithium or sodium valproate.

38. A Donepezil

This has a half-life of 70 hours. Galantamine has a half-life of 7–8 hours. Rivastigmine has a half-life of 1.5 hours. Tacrine has a half-life of 24–36 hours. Memantine has a half-life of 60–100 hours.

39. C Neutropenia

This is an idiosyncratic reaction that is difficult to predict. It is dose independent. About 2.7% of patients treated with clozapine develop neutropenia, whereas approximately 0.8% will develop agranulocytosis. Immune-mediated and direct cytotoxic effects can explain this side effect. The treatment for agranulocytosis is to stop clozapine. Another example of an idiosyncratic side effect of an antipsychotic medication is neuroleptic malignant syndrome.

40. A Anorexia nervosa

Normal limits for QTc are <440 ms for men and <470 ms for women. There is a strong evidence that a QTc interval >500 ms is associated with a risk of arrhythmia. Hypokalaemia, hypomagnesaemia, hypocalcaemia, long QT syndrome, bradycardia, ischaemic heart disease, myocarditis, myocardial infarction, left ventricular hypertrophy, extreme physical exertion, stress or shock, anorexia nervosa, extremes of age (children and elderly people) and female gender are risk factors for QTc prolongation and arrhythmia.

41. D Simpson–Angus scale

This patient has extrapyramidal side effects due to the use of a depot antipsychotic medication. The Simpson–Angus scale is widely used in clinical trials of antipsychotic drugs to assess extrapyramidal symptoms. It is relatively easy to administer in a clinical setting. The brief psychiatric rating scale is used to rate psychiatric symptoms rather than motor side effects. The Bush Francis scale is used to rate catatonic features. The Barnes' akathisia rating scale is used to assess akathisia. The unified Parkinson's disease rating scale is used to assess Parkinson's disease, not drug-induced parkinsonism.

42. D Mirtazapine

Depression is seen in about 30–40% of patients who survive a stroke. Mirtazapine, nortriptyline, fluoxetine, escitalopram and sertraline are recommended for prophylaxis. SSRIs, nortriptyline and mirtazapine are recommended to treat post-stroke depression. If a patient is prescribed warfarin, citalopram is the recommended SSRI due to fewer drug interactions. When using SSRI in an anticoagulated or aspirin-treated patient, use of a proton pump inhibitor should be considered for gastric protection.

43. C Pregabalin

All of the drugs mentioned are antiepileptic medication. Pregabalin is also licensed for the treatment of generalised anxiety disorder. In addition gabapentin and pregabalin are licensed for neuropathic pain and indicated in conditions such as fibromyalgia. Lamotrigine is also licensed for prophylaxis of bipolar depression. Vigabatrin and tiagabine are usually used as an adjunct treatment for epilepsy.

44. D Stop lithium and continue haloperidol

Lithium is best avoided in the first trimester because of its teratogenic potential. Antipsychotics (preferably first generation, but now evidence is building up for second-generation antipsychotics) should be used as mood stabilisers in pregnancy, if required. This patient is at high risk of relapse if the medications are stopped. There is no need to switch to chlorpromazine. Switching unnecessarily is associated with a risk of relapse.

45. B John Kane

Table 1.2 describes the contribution of key people in psychiatry.

Table 1.2 Famous people and their contribution to psychiatry

Name	Contribution
John Cade	Discovered mood-stabiliser effects of lithium carbonate
John Kane	In 1988, John Kane and colleagues conducted a double-blind study comparing the efficacy of chlorpromazine and clozapine/clozaril in treatment-resistant schizophrenia and established that clozapine was clearly superior to chlorpromazine
Jean Delay and Pierre Deniker	Established antipsychotic effect of the first antipsychotic, chlorpromazine, in the 1950s
Max Fink	Best known for his work on electroconvulsive therapy
Nancy Andreasen	Known figure in use of neuroimaging in the study of schizophrenia

46. D Its use with alcohol can cause hypotension

Alcohol is metabolised by alcohol dehydrogenase, which is further metabolised by aldehyde dehydrogenase. Disulfiram irreversibly inhibits aldehyde dehydrogenase, leading to accumulation of aldehyde in the system, producing symptoms such as flushing, nausea, vomiting and hypotension. It should be used after at least 24 hours of the last alcohol ingestion to avoid any possible disulfiram and alcohol reaction.

47. E Oxazepam

Longer-acting benzodiazepines are likely to be accumulated in the body if liver functions are impaired. It may lead to benzodiazepine toxicity. Therefore, shorter-acting benzodiazepines are preferred such as oxazepam (lorazepam). Diazepam and chlordiazepoxide are drugs of choice for detoxification in normal liver functions. Carbamazepine is used for alcohol detoxification in some countries, but in the presence of liver damage, its use is not recommended. Clonazepam is a longer-acting benzodiazepine.

48. E Telophase

Mitosis and meiosis are two forms of cell division that occur in eukaryotes. Many of the somatic cells go through cell division via the process of mitosis, which is a form of nuclear division. Meiosis is a special form of cell division for sexual reproduction. Mitosis consists of the following stages:

1. **Interphase:** before a cell enters into mitosis it goes into a growth period called interphase.
2. **Prophase:** it is a stage in which chromatin condenses into chromosomes.
3. **Metaphase:** it is a stage in which chromosomes get aligned on metaphase plate.
4. **Anaphase:** in this stage paired chromosomes separate and move to the opposite ends of the cell.
5. **Telophase:** it is in this stage that division of the cytoplasm begins.

49. C mRNA

Postmortem examination for gene expression studies are challenging due to problems with variability in intactness of RNA and biological variants. Intact RNA is essential for these studies to be carried out appropriately. Several studies have concluded that mRNA is stable in postmortem human brain and hence can be used for gene expression. Stability of RNA in postmortem tissue differs with the tissue type and also the tissue storage conditions.

50. E Twin adoption study

There has always been a debate about the role of nature and nurture in human development. Twin and adoption studies are the methods of choice for finding out relative contribution of both gene and environment on development. Adoption studies largely consider the impact of environment on the development of a child who has been adopted into a family. Heritability is described as what proportion of observed trait in individuals is due to genetic differences. It is mainly studied by conduction family and twin studies. A family study is conducted basically to answer the question: 'Is the phenotype familial?' Linkage analysis answers the question, 'Where the genes located?' Association analysis helps to find out, 'what the responsible genes are.'

51. D Transcription

It is the first step of gene expression in which information from the DNA molecule is transcribed onto an RNA transcript. This process takes place in the nucleus of the cell and consists of five steps: preinitiation, initiation, promoter clearance, elongation and termination. Translation is the process of making proteins from the RNA molecule and takes place in the cytoplasm with the help of ribosomes. Replication, as the name suggests, is a process in which the DNA or genetic material produces a duplicate copy of itself. Modification is a change in phenotype, which is influenced by environmental factors and is not a heritable trait.

52. B It is a ratio of genetic variance to phenotypic variance

Heritability is measured by concordance rate among twin pairs. It is ratio of genetic variance to phenotypic variance ($h_2 = V_g/V_p$), where h^2 is heritability and V_g is genetic variance and V_p is the phenotypic variance. A heritability of 1 will indicate that all the phenotypic variability is due to genetic variance. The proportion of proband twins who have an affected co-twin is called probandwise concordance rate and the proportion of twins where both are affected with the disorder is called pairwise concordance rate.

53. D Linkage analysis

Genetic linkage is described as investigating the co-segregation of the disease and a set of genetic markers while studying disease in families. The aim of linkage analysis is to determine the location of the gene(s) on a chromosome for a trait of interest, e.g. a common disease. A number of genetic disorders associated with intellectual disability are associated with chromosomal rearrangements such as Down's syndrome (trisomy 21), and the phenotype seems to arise because of the loss (e.g. monosomy) or addition (e.g. trisomy) of dosage-sensitive genes of unrelated functions. While studying population genetics, the term used to describe the non-random association of alleles at two or more loci, which might or might not be on the same chromosome, is called linkage disequilibrium. Genomic rearrangement is described as major changes in the size of the DNA from a few hundred base-pairs to megabases by processes such as deletion, insertion, translocation, duplication and other mutational changes. The gene dosage effect refers to the number of gene copies that are present in a cell or nucleus.

54. B Genetic association analysis

In linkage analysis, random DNA markers (consisting of DNA polymorphism) are used as proxies for any nearby risk genes. However, to determine if a particular or specific gene variant is directly affecting the risk for the disorder, or is very tightly linked to such a gene, the most appropriate method is genetic association analysis.

55. B Markers will not undergo recombination and will be inherited together

Genes that are tightly located near each other on a chromosome tend to be inherited together on meiosis during gene expression. These gene markers are inherited together without undergoing recombination and hence are termed 'genetically linked'. The logarithm of odds (LOD) score is a method used in linkage analysis to determine the frequency of recombination. The LOD score of −2 or less excludes linkage at that particular value of recombinant fraction and that a LOD of 3+ indicates 1000 to 1 odds that the linkage observed is not by chance.

56. A For association studies, the DNA marker has to be in the disease gene itself

Genetic association studies are used to find out if there is a correlation between a disease and genetic variation. It is used to identify the candidate gene that may have played a role in a particular disease. A DNA marker has to be in the disease gene itself or very tightly linked to it. In linkage analysis, linkage can be detected between the markers over large distances. The linkage analysis can be used to 'scan the genome'. Mutation analysis of polymorphisms is carried out by association analysis. It is popular in clinical and genetic counselling settings. There is documented evidence that there is an association between the human leukocyte antigen system and several diseases, such as type 1 diabetes mellitus and multiple sclerosis. The power of association is related directly to the quantitative trait locus (QTL) heritability, whereas the power of linkage is more closely related to the square of the QTL heritability.

57. B Most genes encode peptides and are transcribed by RNA polymerase 2

Expression of genetic information is unidirectional from DNA to RNA to polypeptides, and involves transcription which is in 5′-3′ orientation. Only one strand acts as a template called template/antisense strand, and the other strand as non-template/sense strand. In the process of transcription, three RNA polymerases (1, 2 and 3) including transcriptional factors are involved. RNA splicing, capping and polyadenylation are post-transcriptional. They occur in the nucleus and involve the mRNA. This is then followed by translation, wherein mRNA is transported from the nucleus into the cytoplasm and translation occurs in ribosomes by using tRNA. Messenger RNA has a codon and tRNA has anticodons that are complementary to each other. This leads to production of polypeptides. In most cases, the initiation codon is AUG; mRNA continues to be translated until a termination codon has been reached. There are many amino acids that need several codons for their expression whereas tryptophan and methionine are specified by a single codon. There is post-translational modification including methylation, phosphorylation and other.

58. B Fragile X syndrome

This syndrome is the second most common specific cause of learning disability after Down's syndrome, although it is the most common inherited cause for learning disability. It accounts for 10% of learning disability. It is usually of mild to moderate in severity. Its clinical features include enlarged testes, large ears, long face and flat feet. Gaze aversion is a striking feature in affected males. There is CGG trinucleotide repeat in the fragile X mental retardation-1 (*FMR1*) gene present at a fragile site at Xq27.3, and this is the cytogenetic marker. Around 1% of children with autistic disorder have fragile X syndrome and 30% of fragile X syndrome patients have autistic features.

59. B Respiratory perturbations

Perturbation or disturbance in respiration has been most convincingly linked to panic disorder in adults. It is shown to aggregate in families and increases familial risk of panic disorder. However, in children, respiratory perturbations are associated with separation anxiety disorder.

60. E Serotonin

One of the most robust findings in autism research has been an increased level of peripheral serotonin in a third of children with autism. Recent studies have identified a candidate gene for autism known as *CELF6*. Mutation in this gene is associated with a decrease in levels of serotonin and autism-like symptoms. Possible involvement of dopamine is indicated by the presence of stereotypy motions in autism.

61. D 60:40

In a landmark study by Kendler and colleagues on twins, the percentage ratio of direct:indirect effects of genetic liability to depression are 60:40 respectively. The direct effect is a result of the genes transmitted in the family, whereas the indirect effect is largely mediated by stressful events, neuroticism and a past history of depression.

62. B 35%

Numerous studies in family, twin and adopted children have identified the role of genetics and heritability in eating disorders. The concordance rate for anorexia nervosa is 55% in monozygotic twins and 5% in dizygotic twins. The concordance rates in bulimia nervosa for monozygotic and dizygotic twins are 35% and 30% respectively, suggesting that the genetic component is much more important in heritability of anorexia nervosa than bulimia nervosa.

63. E Penetrance

The probability of expression of an allele when present in the genotype is termed 'penetrance'. For example, if 5 out of 10 individuals with the allele express the respective trait, the trait is said to be 50% penetrant. Even when the allele is present, all phenotypes that are expressed will not be manifested to the fullest degree (penetrance 100%), which indicates that even when the allele is present its expression is variable. In medical genetics, it is a term used to describe the likelihood of the allele resulting in the disease. Depending on the degree of penetrance, it can be complete, highly penetrant, incomplete or low penetrant. Ascertainment is a sampling bias possibility in twin studies that can affect the outcomes. This bias can be overcome by using a population-based sample.

64. C Neuroticism

Suicidal behaviour can have a genetic predisposition and certain candidate endophenotypes can influence suicide risk. Some studies have suggested that this genetic predisposition to suicide risk may be independent of mental illness-related risk. Certain personality traits such as impulsivity, aggression and neuroticism are linked to suicide risk. The impulsive–aggressive continuum is related to serotoninergic dysfunction whereas neuroticism is related to γ-aminobutyric acid type A and serotonin dysfunction. Neuropsychological endophenotypes such as decision-making and executive functions also influence the risk of suicide. Changes in the amygdala and prefrontal cortex metabolism are other candidate endophenotypes related to suicide risk.

65. A Cerebrospinal fluid 5-hydroxyindoleacetic acid A levels

Changes in CSF 5-HIAA levels have been associated with impulsive suicide attempts. This indicates a central serotoninergic dysfunction that is due to a *TPH2* gene polymorphism.

66. C Low voltage alpha activity

Two kinds of EEG activities are used as endophenotypes in alcohol dependence. Low-voltage α activity has been noticed in healthy non-alcohol-dependent volunteers but who have a positive family history of alcohol dependence. β Waves have been noticed to be different in alcohol dependent patients compared with controls.

67. A Behavioural disturbances in childhood are associated with higher rates of alcoholism

Conduct disorder and behavioural disturbances in childhood lead to higher rates of alcoholism. Studies have shown that alcoholic males with a family history of alcoholism have a greater severity of alcoholism and poorer outcomes than those with a negative family history. Earlier age of onset, <15 years of age at first drink, is associated with increased rates of alcoholism and substance misuse. Children of alcoholic parents are likely to face poor parenting and are exposed to high-risk environments. They have poor performance in school and their occupation. The rates of familial alcoholism are high among poor socioeconomic categories.

68. D Chromosomal variations in chromosome 4 are strongly related to alcoholism

A study in Irish affected sibling pairs of alcohol dependence is a linkage study analysing the genetic aspects of alcohol misuse. The results of the study indicate a strong linkage for a number of alcohol dependence criteria to a broad region of chromosome 4. There was also weak linkage to several other regions including 1q44, 13q31 and 22q11, 2q37, 9q21, 9q34 and 18 p11 for alcohol dependence syndrome.

69. B Autism

Genetic predisposition relates to how high the risk of occurrence of a disease is in relatives. The strongest effect for genetic predisposition is seen in autism and attention deficit hyperactivity disorder (ADHD). It is approximately 50-fold in autism and ADHD, 10-fold in schizophrenia, and 5-fold in anxiety and unipolar depression. Heritability of bipolar affective disorder is 85%, schizophrenia 83% and unipolar depression in females and males 42% and 29%, respectively. The concordance rate for anorexia nervosa in monozygotic twins is 40% and in dizygotic twins 15%.

70. C CREB

CREB is an abbreviation for cAMP-response element-binding protein. It is a transcription factor implicated in wide range of psychiatric conditions. There are studies showing a strong link between CREB activities and alcohol- and substance-seeking behaviour. Regulation of CREB activity could be the mode of action of lithium as well as antidepressants.

71. E Individuals with the COMT gene *val/val* allele are at high risk of developing cannabis-induced psychosis

Allelic variation in the COMT gene is associated with an increased incidence of psychosis related to cannabis misuse. Individuals who had *val* allele were at high risk of developing psychosis compared with individuals who had the *met* allele. Cannabis misuse can cause psychosis in certain individuals and is irreversible in many. Dunedin studies have shown that individuals who give a history of psychotic experiences and use cannabis at age 11 years are associated with increased incidence of psychosis at age 26 years.

72. B The environmental factors that predispose as well as trigger psychiatric disorders

Anthony, Eaton and Henderson coined the term 'environment'. It refers to the totality of equivalent environmental influences and includes predisposing factors such as intrauterine exposure to radiation, teratogens, family income and neighbourhoods, as well as provoking environmental factors that can act as a trigger of psychiatric disorders, such as social stressors and crisis in personal relationships.

73. B Chromosome 22

Deletions on the end of chromosome 22 cause a wide range of physical as well as mental health abnormalities. This includes psychosis that is indistinguishable from schizophrenia.

74. A The ecological and social settings that an individual shares with parents

An ontogenetic niche, described by West and King, means that an organism shares not only genes but also the ecological and social environment with its parents. Nature (genes) and nurture (ecological and social setting) are both important in the overall development of an offspring. They work hand in hand. Sometimes, it is said that nature loads the gun and nurture fires it!

75. A Environmental factors play a more important role in the development of depression than genetic factors

When family studies into first-degree relatives conclude that there is increased incidence of illness in first-degree relatives, all it tells us is that the illness is familial. This could be due to genetic or shared environmental factors. If the study is extended to second- and third-degree relatives then it can provide significant information. If the findings show that there is increased risk of developing depression in parents, siblings and offspring as probands, whereas second- and third-degree relatives do not have the increased risk, this means that environmental factors play a more important role in the development of depression than genetic factors.

76. C 1 in 10

European study of epidemiology of mental disorders (ESEMED) is a multicentric study conducted in six European countries such as Belgium, France, Netherlands, Spain, Italy and Germany. This study is a part of WHO mental health survey initiative. According to ESEMED, the life time prevalence of mental disorders in Europe is 1 in 4 whereas the prevalence of mental disorder in the past 1 year (12-month prevalence) is 1 in 10.

77. B 2–4 years

The study of Zanarini et al. (2007) noted two main findings: out of the 24 symptoms studied over a 10-year period < 15% were exhibited; the other 12 symptoms declined less substantially with about 20–40% still exhibiting at the end of the 10-year period.

78. B 1–5%

The reported prevalence of elderly people in the community with paraphrenia is 0.1–4%. According to Targun and Abbott (1999), the prevalence is 0.2–4.7%. Hence, one can safely assume a prevalence of 1–5% as the right answer in this case.

79. B 10%

Approximately 10% of the elderly population admitted to a psychiatric ward have paraphrenia. Studies suggest that a wide range, from 10% to 63%, of the elderly population in nursing homes have psychotic symptoms.

80. B 5 years

If the onset of dementia is delayed by 5 years, the prevalence can be reduced by 50%. A delay of 6 months can also reduce prevalence by 6%. This delay can be achieved by successful risk reduction strategies.

81. C 10%

Ritchie et al (2010) concluded that elimination of depression from the elderly population can lead to a mean reduction of 10.3% in new cases of dementia over a period of 7 years. In addition, if depression and diabetes are eliminated from the elderly population and there is an increase in fruit and vegetable consumption, there can be a mean reduction of 20.7% in new cases of dementia. Of note is that depression was found to make the biggest contribution.

82. C Prevalence of 10–15%

Problem behaviours in patients with learning disability are commoner in males in the age group 15–34 years. The prevalence is about 10–15%. The prevalence increases with an increase in the severity of the learning difficulty. The problem behaviours tend to be of more than one type and include demanding behaviour, verbal and physical aggression, destructiveness and self-injury. These behaviours are usually long standing.

83. A Early onset is associated with poor prognosis

Alcohol is responsible for 10% of the dementia population. It may contribute to 21–24% of cognitive impairment in mid-adulthood. The frequency of alcohol-related dementia is higher in socioeconomically deprived areas and most of the cases present at age 50–60 years. The earlier the onset of alcohol-related dementia the poorer the prognosis. The prevalence of the Wernicke–Korsakoff syndrome due to thiamine deficiency is on the rise.

84. C First rank symptoms at the baseline

Possible predictors of course and outcome in schizophrenia are sociodemographic status, initial clinical state, treatment response, history of past psychotic episodes and treatment, premorbid personality, functioning, type of the onset, family history of psychiatric disorders, variables of brain morphology and neurocognition. Good prognosis is indicated in acute onset, prominent affective features, no family history, paranoid subtype, good premorbid adjustment and older age of onset.

85. B It can explore multiple outcomes and exposures

Cross-sectional studies are simplest of all individual-level studies. They are cheaper and quicker than other studies and can explore multiple outcomes and exposures at the same time. They are used to quantify the prevalence of the disease in question. It allows for hypothesis generation based on the aetiology. It does have some limitations such as researcher and recall bias. It is not a feasible study design for rare diseases and does not establish a temporal association.

86. D It is useful to generate a hypothesis

A qualitative study helps in generating a hypothesis. This study is concerned with an individual's personal meanings, experiences, feelings, values and other types of opinions. Qualitative study uses passive observation, participant observation, in-depth interviews and focus groups. The sampling method used is theoretical and is analysed by inductive reasoning and validity.

87. E 60%

According to the WHO, suicide rates have increased by 60% in the last 45 years. The global mortality rate is 16 per 100,000 or one death every 40 seconds.

88. A 15–44 years; males

In the UK from 2000 to 2009, the suicide rate was found to be highest among males aged 15–44 years.

89. E Point prevalence

Prevalence and incidence are two measures of disease frequency.

Point prevalence is the number of individuals with the disease in a population at a particular point in time. It is expressed as a proportion. Period prevalence is the number of individuals with the disease in a population over a period of time. It is expressed as a rate. Life-time prevalence is the proportion of individuals who have or have had a given disease.

90. D Low incidence, long duration of illness

Prevalence is defined as a proportion of the product of the incidence rate and average duration of a disease.

Prevalence = Incidence × Duration of illness.

Hence, prevalence can be high even if incidence is low due to a long duration of illness.

91. A Cumulative incidence

Cumulative incidence or incidence risk is the number of new cases of a disease over a period of time out of the total population at risk.

Incidence density or incidence rate is the number of new cases of a disease over a period of time out of the total person-time of observation.

92. E Standardised mortality ratio

The number of deaths observed divided by number of expected deaths multiplied by 100 gives the standardised mortality rate (SMR). An SMR of 100 signifies that the standard population and population under study have the same mortality rate. If the 95% CI of SMR exceeds '1' it is considered statistically significant.

93. A Beck's depression inventory

Rating scales used in psychiatry can be self-administered, semi-structured or clinician administered. Beck's depression inventory and Zung's self-rating depression scale are self-administered. The brief psychiatric rating scale, clinical global improvement scale, hamilton's rating scale for depression, Yale–Brown–compulsive scale are all scales that are used for rating symptom severity and change in a mental illness. These scales are administered by clinicians.

94. D To monitor the response to treatment

The Yale–Brown obsessive compulsive scale (Y-BOCS) gives a measure of distress and not anxiety. It is not a diagnostic tool and is used only to assess the severity of the obsessive–compulsive disorder. It is this property of Y-BOCS that is made use of while monitoring the progress of the patient in response to the treatment. It is extensively used in clinical settings. There are 10 questions, 5 for obsessions and 5 for compulsion, and all are rated on a Likert scale with a minimum total score of 0 and a maximum of 40. A score of 0–7 is subclinical, 8–15 mild, 16–23 moderate, 24–31 severe and 32–40 extreme.

95. D Halo effect

This effect is a cognitive bias in which there is a tendency to overestimate a response by a rater based on previous impressions, assumptions and judgements. It was termed 'halo effect' by psychologist Edward Thorndike. The Hawthorne effect is an effect whereby patients modify their behaviour just because they are participating in an experimental study. The ceiling effect is when the dependent measure puts an artificially low ceiling on how high a person may score; it can lead to an undesirable outcome. Ecological fallacy is an error of deduction that involves deriving conclusions about individuals just on the basis of an analysis of group data. Central limit theorem: as sample size increase, the sample mean will approach a normal distribution.

96. C 100,000 live births

The maternal mortality rate is the number of maternal deaths per 100,000 live births in the same time period. Maternal death is the death of a woman while pregnant or within 42 days of termination of pregnancy. This does not take into account the duration and site of the pregnancy, any complication or its management. However, it does take accidents and incidental cause into account. Pregnancy-related death is defined as the death of a woman while pregnant or within 42 days of termination of pregnancy, irrespective of the cause of death.

97. E Unless rehearsed, storage in short-term memory is limited to 30 seconds

Transfer of memory into long-term store begins immediately when information enters short-term store. Short-term memory is also known as 'primary' or 'working' memory whereas long-term memory is also known as secondary memory. Encoding is related to concepts of information processing and attention. Unless rehearsed, storage in short-term memory is limited to no more than 30 seconds, with a capacity of around seven units. Theoretically, long-term memory is permanent and has unlimited capacity.

98. E Neurocognitive impairments usually begin after first episode of schizophrenia

Neurocognitive impairments are reliably and broadly present in the first episode of schizophrenia. Larger IQ impairments are seen in the first episode compared with later stages. Patients with schizophrenia demonstrate cognitive impairments that range from mild to severe. These impairments are due to neither poor motivation nor the presence of psychotic symptoms. They usually remain stable over time and include deficits in perceptual skills, motor skills, verbal skills, selective attention, spatial and verbal working memory, verbal learning, non-verbal memory, procedural memory, long-term factual memory and executive functions. These impairments are central features of schizophrenia as suggested by their presence before the diagnosis is made.

99. E The trait approach to personality assessment is the basis for the ICD-10 classification.

The informants in personality assessments should have a good knowledge of the person for a number of years. The current assessments of personality, as well as the ICD-10 and DSM-IV classifications, are based on the measurement of traits although this method is of questionable reliability. There are objective and projective personality assessments. An example of an objective personality assessment is the Minnesota multiphasic personality inventory (MMPI). The most researched personality inventory is the MMPI.

100. B Personality disorder is commonly observed among the perpetrators

According to the WHO, there are five types of child maltreatments.

1. Physical abuse
2. Sexual abuse
3. Emotional abuse
4. Exploitation
5. Neglect.

The definitions used by the Government in England and Wales are similar to those used by the WHO, although there may be operational differences. Fabricated or induced illness is a form of child maltreatment more than parental psychopathology, although observations suggest high rates of personality disorder among the observers. The child is harmed directly or indirectly, leading to a variety of presentations.

101. D Puberty lasts longer than in the previous generations

The age of reaching puberty has decreased in the western population from 17 years to below 12–13 years. The average age of menarche in Britain is 12 years and 10 months. One in six girls reaches puberty before the age of 8 years and one in fourteen 8-year-old boys have pubic hair. Puberty starts earlier and lasts longer according to the children of the 1990s' study conducted by Bristol University's Institute of Child Health. It is noticed that boys also mature earlier.

102. E 40%

Thomas et al (1968) conducted a study of temperament in infants in the 1950s. Data was gathered initially by parental interviews that looked at nine traits that were combined to describe three temperament types.

Table 1.3 Types of temperament		
Temperament	**Percentage in cohort**	**Description**
Easy	40	Playful, regular patterns of eating and sleeping, adapted easily to new situations
Difficult	10	Irritable with irregular eating and sleeping patterns. Responded negatively to new situations
Slow to warm	15	Relatively inactive and tends to withdraw from new situations

The remaining 35% of children could not be placed in any one group.

103. C Non-negotiable parents who are strict

There are three main parenting styles described. An authoritarian parenting style is where parents do not negotiate and are strict. The boundaries set are clear and rigid. The children tend to have low self-esteem and can be socially withdrawn. An authoritative parenting style is where parents discuss and explain to the child so that there are firm rules with shared decision-making. The children are usually sociable and popular and have a positive self-esteem. A permissive parenting style is where there are few limits set by the parents with no clear guidelines and the children usually have poor impulse control and display aggression.

104. B Child experiences maternal deprivation

According to Bowlby, if a child before the age of 1 year is separated from the mother when she is working, maternal deprivation is likely to occur. Rarely, privation, where no attachment is formed, may occur. Separation anxiety may develop. Object permanence development will not be affected. The strange situation test is an inappropriate test because the child may not respond when the mother returns as a sign of self-reliance rather than avoidance. This occurs because the child is used to separation.

105. D Studies use it in the context of intergenerational transfer of attachment patterns

The adult attachment interview is a structured interview that explores an individual's experience of attachment relationships in childhood. There are four possible attachment styles such as:

1. Secure/autonomous
2. Dismissive
3. Preoccupied/entangled
4. Unresolved/disorganised.

Studies mainly use it in the context of intergenerational transfer of attachment patterns or intergenerational continuity. In summary, people parent their children as they were parented.

106. D The paranoid–depressive positions are never fully resolved in adult life

The work with regard to paranoid and depressive positions was led primarily by Melanie Klein. In this case, an infant divides the caregiver into an external object that is all good or an internal object that is all bad. This includes two stages known as the depressive position and the paranoid–schizoid position. Projection, splitting and projective identification are the primitive defence mechanisms observed in the paranoid–schizoid position.

107. E Winnicot

Winnicot proposed the following concepts:

- Holding environment indicates that, for appropriate development in a child, a parent needs to hold them physically and psychologically.
- Good-enough mother is a mother who needs to be responsive but not extreme, as in too responsive or unresponsive, to ensure adequate emotional development in the infant.
- Countertransference hate means that parents, like infants, can bring strong emotions to their care such as hate, which needs to be addressed.

108. E More than one dream idea is combined into a single mental image

A dream, according to Freud, is the fulfilment of a wish. Manifest content refers to what we are aware of upon waking. Dream interpretation is the process of making sense of the manifest content of dreams by 'translating' it. In dream work, the latent content, the 'underlying wish', is changed into manifest content and involves displacement, condensation and concrete representation. Displacement is the dream content that substitutes the target of one's feelings onto another person. Condensation is more than one dream's idea combined into a single mental image. Concrete representation is an abstract concept, revealed in a concrete way and is sometimes called dramatisation.

109. C The symptoms may symbolise the wish with which they are linked

Neurotic symptoms are viewed as similar to dreams. Dreams are considered to be the 'royal road to unconsciousness'. The symptoms are felt to be the expression of an unconscious and may symbolise the wish to which it is linked. The symptom is usually physical and the cause mental.

110. B Appropriate roles or goals are abandoned because they are perceived as forbidden or dangerous

Cognitive–analytical therapy was devised by Anthony Ryle for use in the UK National Health Service. Three different patterns of unrevisable, maladaptive procedures called traps, dilemmas and snags are described.

Traps are negative assumptions that generate acts which produce consequences that reinforce the assumptions. Dilemmas are brought about by the person acting as though the available actions or roles are limited to only polarised alternatives (false dichotomies). Snags occur when the appropriate roles or goals are abandoned because the individual makes an assumption that others would oppose, or because they are perceived as forbidden or dangerous.

111. B Displacement

Defence mechanisms are unconscious ways of dealing with experiences. Denial occurs when the individual does not acknowledge an aspect of reality. Displacement is shifting of the emotion from the real target onto a substitute. Humour is where comedy is used to manage the emotions that arise and express them. Reaction formation is where the individual expresses the opposite of what is felt or thought. In sublimation, an individual channels the emotions towards a socially positive substituted activity.

112. A It has four basic functions

According to Jung there are three levels that make up the psyche such as consciousness, personal unconscious and collective unconscious. The consciousness has four basic functions, namely thinking, feeling, sensing and intuiting. The personal unconscious which is made up of an individual's unique experiences involving repression is accessible through recall. The collective unconscious is where the mind has inherited characteristics that influence how one reacts and the type of experiences these will be. This includes archetypes that are representational images with symbolic meaning.

113. A Expression of affect in a supportive environment

According to Yalom the following are descriptions of the therapeutic process that occur in group work:

- Universality: where members recognise that the experiences are common and can link them to those that occur in society.
- Corrective recapitulation of the primary family experience: patients repeat childhood experiences in their family with the group, without their knowledge.
- Imitative behaviour: individuals improve their interactions in the group by modelling other's helpful behaviours of communication and listening.
- Interpersonal learning: gives feedback on how they are seen by others.
- Catharsis: when the individual feels unburdened difficult emotions, by expressing affect in a supportive environment.
- Group cohesiveness: members have a sense of being incorporated with others.
- Imparting of information: learning from others relating to their difficulties.
- Instillation of hope: seeing other members improve.
- Development of socialising techniques: members enhance their socialising skills through the supportive environment.
- Existential factors: encouraged to take responsibility for one's thoughts, feelings and actions.
- Self-understanding: develop a deeper understanding of the self with regard to their interactions with other members.
- Altruism: improving one's self-esteem as members learn that they can help each other.

114. B Members of the family are 'prescribed' their symptom which can paradoxically lead to an alteration

The following techniques are used in systemic family therapy:

- **In-session, structural interventions:** different positions are assigned to parts of the family structure.
- **Paradoxical injunction:** members of the family are 'prescribed' their symptom which can paradoxically lead to an alteration.
- **Reciprocity negotiation:** practical solutions are developed between family members.
- **Homework:** tasks are assigned to family members to complete between sessions; these involve a change in their actions to see how it affects the system.
- **Adjust to the symptom:** thought is given to how to live with symptoms if they cannot be altered.

115. E Systemic family therapy

This is the treatment of choice for adolescents with anorexia nervosa and is particularly effective with early onset anorexia. By the end of therapy, >50% reach a healthy weight'. 60–90% of patients with anorexia recover completely, with only 10–15% continuing to be seriously ill. It is included in the NICE guideline recommendations under psychological interventions.

The different systemic approaches developed include:

- Structural
- Strategic
- Milan systemic
- Narrative
- Psychoeducational
- Behavioural.

The structural approach looks at the family structure; it considers this as the family structure with generational hierarchies and semipermeable boundaries important for family function. Strategic systemic therapy is based on the hypothesis that behaviours that aim to suppress the symptoms in turn maintain it. The Milan systemic approach has changed over the years from the style of using paradoxical questioning to that of reflexive and circular questioning. The technique focuses on questioning various family members about their relationships. Narrative therapy involves helping families to create stories as a means of interpreting events. The psychoeducational approach combines behavioural and structural techniques. The behavioural approach uses techniques to maximise the positive and minimise the negative through goal setting, contingency contracting and operant conditioning.

116. B Cognitive–behavioural therapy

As recommended by the NICE guidelines, CBT is recommended as a psychological intervention in depression as well as for a variety of other presentations. There are randomised controlled trials to support its use. It is considered to be a short-term, problem-focused, psychosocial intervention and does not aim to achieve major personality change. It explores and works on the inter-relationship between one's thoughts, feelings, physiological reactions and behaviours.

There are three main areas of dysfunction identified in CBT such as conditional assumptions, negative automatic thoughts and core beliefs

117. C Excessive responsibility

In cognitive therapy, the cognitive errors derived from assumptions include the following:

- Assuming temporal causality: if it was true in the past then it will always be true
- Catastrophising: always think the worst and then it will happen
- Dichotomous thinking: things are viewed as extremes, either bad or good
- Excessive responsibility: assume personal responsibility for all negative outcomes
- Over-generalising: if it happens at one time then it will happen in all cases
- Selective abstraction: attention is given only to failure and negative outcomes
- Self-references: my bad performance is the centre of everyone's attention.

118. B It was developed by Linehan

Dialectic behavioural therapy (DBT) is an integrative therapy developed by Marsha Linehan. It is beneficial in individuals with borderline personality disorder. DBT involves group and individual interventions with social skills training, mindfulness and mediation. It is an intensive therapy with weekly and daily sessions that can extend up to 2 years.

119. E Target assessment

Eye movement desensitisation and reprocessing (EMDR) was developed by Francine Shapiro and is a treatment for post-traumatic stress disorder. There are several stages of EMDR. It begins with history and preparation. During target assessment, the target traumatic memory is explored and defined. Desensitisation is the therapist's directed evocation of the picture, which represents the memory image to desensitise. During installation, the patient is asked to recall the trauma and to hold in mind the preferred positive, and is then treated with repeated sets of eye movements. The next stage is body scan which involves asking the patient to close the eyes and focus on bodily sensations. Finally there is closure and re-evaluation.

Habit reversal training is a behavioural treatment package useful in tics and other obsessive–compulsive spectrum disorders, trichotillomania, nail biting, etc. It has the following components: awareness training, competing response training, contingency management, relaxation training and generalisation training.

120. D Step 4–considered if there is high risk of self-harm

According to the NICE clinical guidance, the following steps should be considered as treatment of generalised anxiety disorder (GAD).

Step 1: it is for identification and assessment in all known and suspected cases of GAD.
Step 2: once diagnosed with GAD, if there is no improvement after education or watching in primary care, low level psychological therapy is considered.
Step 3: if step 2 has failed, a high level of psychological therapy such as CBT and applied relaxation is considered. In addition, medication is considered at this step.
Step 4: if there is high risk of self-harm, self-neglect, failed step 3 or complex GAD condition, then day hospital or inpatient stay can be considered in addition to medication and psychological therapy.

121. E There is a good research base for psychological management for comorbid disorders seen in ASPD

Most of the therapies, when used in the criminal justice system, aim to reduce offending behaviour. These therapies such as behavioural modification, graded exposure, problem-solving techniques and social skills training are largely based on social learning theory. Virtually all interventions delivered in the criminal justice system are aimed at reducing offending behaviour.

122. C Drug treatments have a higher relapse rate than CBT on discontinuation in generalised anxiety disorder

Most trials that have been done with the combination of CBT and medication in mild-to-moderate depression did not show that they were more effective than either alone. Stuart and Bowers (1995) showed, in an inpatient population, that the combination of CBT and antidepressants was more effective than medication alone in those with more severe depression. Evidence suggests that CBT is as effective as antidepressant medication in outpatient depression. The combination of CBT and antidepressant medication may be more effective than either alone in severe depression. After ending treatment, relapse rates of depression are lower with CBT than with antidepressants. Drug treatment has a higher relapse rate than CBT on discontinuation in anxiety.

123. B Debriefing

The National Institute for Health and Care Excellence (NICE) guidance does not recommend debriefing. There is some evidence that this can actually be more harmful. Rose et al (2009) found that psychological debriefing as a control or educational intervention can be worse or at the most equivalent in reducing severity or PTSD. It may even increase the risk of PTSD and depression. There is no evidence to support the routine use of debriefing in PTSD.

124. B Flooding

This occurs in vivo and is also known as implosion. The therapist exposes the patient to a controlled environment to evoke anxiety and no hierarchy is employed. Here the anxiety is generated but the patient is prevented from escaping.

125. B Motivation to change

Group therapy is a therapy in which carefully selected members guided by a therapist help one another to bring about personality change. Membership of a group uses the following inclusion criteria: motivation to change, ability to perform the group task, problem areas compatible with the goals of the group, compatibility with the group norms and ability to tolerate group setting.

126. C Dialectic behavioural therapy

In the NICE guidelines for borderline personality disorder, there is a recommendation to consider dialectic behavioural therapy for women with borderline personality disorder who repeatedly self-harm.

127. B After long-term deprivation children become self-sufficient through detachment

The long-term effect of short-term deprivation is separation anxiety which is also associated with long-term deprivation. Short-term deprivation includes admissions for mother or child into hospital for a period of <3 months. Long-term deprivation follows death and more commonly these days divorce. The effects include detachment, clinging behaviour, oscillation between clinging and detachment, increased aggressive behaviour or psychosomatic reactions.

128. A Being abused as a child

Risk characteristics of parents who abuse children include being a single parent, young age, abused themselves as a child, low self-esteem, unrealistic expectations of the child's development, and inconsistent or punishment-oriented discipline. Risk factors of the environment for child abuse include social isolation, current stress and a large family.

129. A About 60% of couples cohabit before they marry

Couples who cohabit before marriage are less likely to be satisfied by their marriages. About 40% of couples who cohabit do not marry. Married people tend to live longer, are happier and healthier, and have lower rates of mental illnesses than divorced, single or widowed individuals. Divorce rates are highest in the first 5 years of life and then again after 15–25 years of being married. The highest divorce rate in individuals in England and Wales is for those in their late 20s.

130. E Parents have other mental health problems

The presence of the following vulnerability factors in parents can be useful in identifying children at risk of developing conduct problems:

- Parents with other mental health problems
- Parents with substance misuse and/or alcohol problem
- Mother younger than 18 years of age who has a history of being maltreated in childhood
- Parents who were in residential care
- Parents with history of involvement with criminal justice system, either past or present.

131. E There is a statistically significant association between sexual abuse and lifetime diagnosis of sleep disorders

In addition to sleep disorders, sexual abuse is also associated with several other mental disorders such as suicide attempts, depression, eating disorder, PTSD, emotionally unstable personality disorder and anxiety disorders. This association is independent of gender and the age when the abuse occurred. If there is a history of rape, it increases the association of sexual abuse, depression and eating disorder.

Chapter 2

Test questions: 2

Questions: MCQs

For each question, select one answer option.

NEUROSCIENCES: NEUROANATOMY

1. A 52-year-old woman was recently diagnosed with a lesion in her subthalamic nucleus. Which of the following is the most likely effect of this lesion?

   A Bradykinesia
   B Hemiballismus
   C Huntington's disease
   D Parkinsonism
   E Wilson's disease

2. Which of the following cells are the smallest of all neurons in the cerebellum?

   A Basket cells
   B Golgi cells
   C Granule cells
   D Purkinje cells
   E Stellate cells

3. Which of the following statements about the subdivisions of the brain is correct?

   A Central sulcus delineates the border between parietal and temporal lobes
   B Heschl's gyrus delineates the border between temporal and occipital lobes
   C Lateral fissure separates the temporal and frontal lobes
   D Longitudinal fissure separates the cerebellum into left and right hemispheres
   E Parieto-occipital sulcus separates the occipital and parietal cortex on the lateral aspect of hemisphere

4. Which of the following cranial nerves has a pure sensory component?

   A Abducens nerve
   B Facial nerve
   C Hypoglossal nerve
   D Optic nerve
   E Trochlear nerve

5. Which of the following structures is involved in the auditory pathway?

   A Corona radiata
   B Lateral geniculate body
   C Myer's loop
   D Tectum
   E Trapezoid body

6. A 64-year-old man was diagnosed with Parkinson's disease. Which of the following macroscopic changes would be present in the brain?

    A   Changes in the locus ceruleus
    B   Dilatation of the lateral and third ventricles
    C   Marked atrophy of the cerebral cortex
    D   Marked atrophy of the corpus striatum
    E   Small brain with a reduced mass

7. A 84-year-old man died 10 years after a diagnosis of Alzheimer's disease. Which of the following microscopic changes would be seen on postmortem examination of his brain?

    A   Ballooned neurons
    B   Focal neuronal loss
    C   Hirano's bodies in hippocampus
    D   Pick's bodies
    E   Proliferation of cholinergic neurons

8. Which of the following tumours are derived from Schwann cells?

    A   Gliomas
    B   Haemangioblastomas
    C   Pituitary adenomas
    D   Medulloblastomas
    E   Neurilemmomas

9. Which of the following statements about amyloid plaques and neurofibrillary tangles is correct?

    A   Amyloid plaques are intracellular accumulations
    B   Amyloid plaques are soluble, composed of BA4 amyloid
    C   Both are pathognomonic of Alzheimer's dementia
    D   Neurofibrillary tangles are intraneuronal aggregations
    E   Neurofibrillary tangles are dephosphorylated protein

10. Which lesions can be demonstrated by using Bielschowsky's stain?

    A   Amyloid plaques
    B   Huntington's disease inclusions
    C   Lewy bodies
    D   Pick's bodies
    E   Prion deposition

11. Which of the following stages constitute the longest percentage of sleep time in a young adult?

    A   Non-rapid eye movement (NREM) stage1
    B   NREM stage 2
    C   NREM stage 3
    D   NREM stage 4
    E   REM

12. According to Erlanger/Gasser, what is the diameter of Aδ cutaneous temperature and pain afferents?

    A   3 μm
    B   5 μm
    C   8 μm
    D   13 μm
    E   15 μm

13. A normal 38-year-old man had undergone an electroencephalogram (EEG) investigation. He was awake but with his eyes closed. What frequency waves would you expect to see on EEG recordings?

    A 0–4 Hz
    B 4–8 Hz
    C 8–13 Hz
    D 13–24 Hz
    E 24–28 Hz

14. A 58-year-old man was diagnosed with sporadic Creutzfeldt–Jakob disease. Which of the following EEG changes will be seen?

    A 3-Hz spike-and-wave activity
    B Hypsarrhythmia
    C Normal or non-specific EEG
    D Periodic discharge with focal δ activity over temporal lobes
    E Triphasic 1–2 Hz discharge

15. Which of the following is the inotropic receptor?

    A Acetylcholine (muscarinic)
    B Acetylcholine (nicotinic)
    C Dopamine
    D γ-Aminobutyric acid B
    E Serotonin (or 5-HT$_1$)

16. A 45-year-old man was diagnosed with depression. What abnormalities can be noted on hypothalamic–pituitary axis regulation?

    A Decreased cortisol levels
    B Decreased adrenal vasopressin
    C Down-regulation of glucocorticoid receptor
    D Reduced corticotrophin-releasing hormone
    E Reduced size of adrenal glands

NEUROSCIENCES: NEUROCHEMISTRY

17. Which of the following is a peptide neurotransmitter?

    A Cholecystokinin
    B Dopamine
    C Adrenaline
    D Glycine
    E Glutamate

18. Which of the following is a precursor of tryptophan?

    A Adrenaline
    B Acetylcholine
    C Dopamine
    D Noradrenaline
    E Serotonin

19. A 34-year-old man was diagnosed with schizophrenia and had active psychotic symptoms. Which neurochemical changes in the glutamate receptor could be responsible for his psychotic symptoms?

    A   Decreased glutamatergic function at N-methyl-D-aspartate (NMDA)
    B   Decreased glutamatergic function at the AMPA (α-amino-3-hydroxy-5-methyl-4-isoxazolepropionic acid) receptor
    C   Decreased glutamatergic function at kainate receptors
    D   Increased glutamatergic function at NMDA
    E   Increased glutamatergic function at γ-aminobutyric acid

20. Which of the following is the precursor in the synthesis of histamine?

    A   Choline
    B   L-Tryptophan
    C   L-Tyrosine
    D   Dopamine β hydroxylase
    E   Histidine

21. A 70-year-old man was diagnosed with Alzheimer's dementia. What would you expect to see on brain neuroimaging?

    A   Disease in and around the front parietal lobes
    B   Increase in grey matter lesions
    C   Increase in ventricular dilatation of 5% per year
    D   Localised atrophy in the hippocampal area
    E   Reduced medial temporal lobe width at level of brain stem

22. What information can be obtained by using a T1-weighted image on MRI of brain?

    A   Anatomical structures
    B   Brain/cerebrospinal fluid contrast
    C   Definition of soft-tissue pathology
    D   Small infarcts
    E   White matter lesions

23. What ligand is used for dopamine receptors D_2/D_3 in positron emission tomography?

    A   [^{11}C]Hyoscine
    B   [^{11}C]Raclopride
    C   [^{18}F]-Flumazenil
    D   [^{18}F]-Fluorodopa
    E   [^{18}F]-Setoperone

24. Which of the following scans uses a radioactive tracer to measure cerebral functions?

    A   CT
    B   fMRI
    C   MRI
    D   Positron emission tomography
    E   Single photon emission computed tomography

25. MRI magnets are rated in teslas units. What is the usual range of MRI scanners used for clinical purpose?

    A   0.001–003 T
    B   0.01–0.03 T
    C   0.3–2.0 T
    D   2–3 T
    E   3–4 T

PSYCHOPHARMACOLOGY: PHARMACOKINETICS

26. If the estimated glomerular filtration rate is 10–50 mL/min per 1.73 m^2 then what is the maximum dose of prescribed paliperidone tablet?

A   2 mg
B   3 mg
C   4 mg
D   5 mg
E   6 mg

27. Which of the following antipsychotics has the best available evidence for use in patients with moderate-to-severe liver impairment?

A   Aripiprazole
B   Haloperidol
C   Paliperidone
D   Quetiapine
E   Risperidone

PSYCHOPHARMACOLOGY: PHARMACODYNAMICS

28. Which of the following about acamprosate is correct?

A   Antagonist of glutamate receptor
B   Antagonist of 5-HT$_3$
C   Dopamine agonist
D   Inhibit alcohol dehydrogenase
E   Partial agonist of 5-HT$_{1A}$

29. Which of the following drugs blocks the transaminase enzyme that converts γ-aminobutyric acid to glutamate?

A   Barbiturates
B   Benzodiazepine
C   Carbamazepine
D   Phenytoin
E   Sodium valproate

30. Which of the following benzodiazepines has the shortest elimination half-life?

A   Diazepam
B   Lorazepam
C   Nitrazepam
D   Oxazepam
E   Temazepam

31. Which of the following drugs is a partial agonist of dopamine receptors?

A   Amisulpiride
B   Aripiprazole
C   Clobazam
D   Paliperidone
E   Ziprasidone

32. What of the following statements about Paliperidone is correct?

   A   Anticholinergic side effects are common
   B   It acts as an agonist on 5-HT$_{2A}$ receptors
   C   It is a precursor of risperidone
   D   It is also available as a depot injection formulation
   E   It is licensed to be used in bipolar affective disorder as a mood stabiliser in the UK

33. Which of the following drugs reduces the anticoagulant effect of warfarin?

   A   Mirtazepine
   B   Selective serotonin reuptake inhibitors
   C   St John's wort
   D   Sodium valproate
   E   Venlafaxine

34. A 32-year-old woman on contraceptive pills discovered that she was pregnant. Which of the following drugs was she most probably taking along with the pills?

   A   Fluoxetine
   B   Olanzapine
   C   St John's wort
   D   Sodium valproate
   E   Venlafaxine

PSYCHOPHARMACOLOGY: ADVERSE REACTIONS

35. Which of the following antidepressants can be used in patients who are worried about weight gain?

   A   Amitriptyline
   B   Imipramine
   C   Lofepramine
   D   Mianserin
   E   Trazadone

36. Which of the following depot antipsychotic injections is associated with post-injection syndrome?

   A   Fluphenazine decanoate
   B   Flupenthixol decanoate
   C   Risperidal Consta
   D   Pipothiazine palmitate
   E   Olanzapine embonate

37. Which of the following explains hypersalivation due to clozapine?

   A α_1-Receptor antagonism
   B   Extrapyramidal side effects
   C   Impaired deglutition
   D M_3-Receptor blockade
   E M_2-Receptor stimulation

38. What is the minimum dose of paracetamol overdose taken within 24 hours that might give rise to hepatocellular necrosis?

   A   50 mg/kg
   B   100 mg/kg

C   150 mg/kg
D   200 mg/kg
E   250 mg/kg

39. Which of the following statements about risk factors for neuroleptic malignant syndrome (NMS) is correct?

A   Dose of antipsychotics affects the risk
B   Family history of NMS is inversely related to the risk of NMS
C   Women are at lesser risk than men
D   Longer duration of treatment with antipsychotics poses greater risk
E   Slow decrease in dosage of antipsychotics increases the risk

PSYCHOPHARMACOLOGY: THEORIES OF ACTION

40. Which of the following drugs should be withdrawn before starting venlafaxine?

A   Duloxetine
B   Mirtazapine
C   Reboxetine
D   Sertraline
E   Trazadone

41. What is the approximate dose of clozapine required for treatment-resistant schizophrenia in a female patient who smokes excessively?

A   300 mg
B   350 mg
C   400 mg
D   450 mg
E   500 mg

42. How many milligrams of valproic acid is equivalent to 500 mg of sodium valproate?

A   100 mg
B   250 mg
C   400 mg
D   433 mg
E   538.2 mg

43. A 65-year-old woman with a history of ischaemic heart disease was noted to be depressed after a recent myocardial infarction. What would be the most appropriate antidepressant to start?

A   Fluoxetine
B   Imipramine
C   Paroxetine
D   Sertraline
E   Venlafaxine

44. Which antiepileptic drug was reported to improve drinking behaviour?

A   Carbamazepine
B   Gabapentin
C   Lamotrigine
D   Sodium valproate
E   Topiramate

45. A 43-year-old man dependent on 20 mg temazepam every day attended the drug and alcohol service with the aim of stopping it. The consultant wanted to convert temazepam to an equivalent dose of diazepam. What is the dose of diazepam prescribed that is equivalent to temazepam 20 mg?

    A   2 mg
    B   5 mg
    C   10 mg
    D   20 mg
    E   40 mg

GENETICS: CELLULAR AND MOLECULAR GENETICS

46. What is the mechanism of production of duplicate DNA copies from template DNA called?

    A   Modification
    B   Replication
    C   Synapsis
    D   Transcription
    E   Translation

47. Which of the following chromosomes is largest in size?

    A   Chromosome 1
    B   Chromosome 2
    C   Chromosome 3
    D   X chromosome
    E   Y chromosome

48. In which of the following phases of cell cycle does DNA synthesis occur?

    A   M phase
    B   G1 phase
    C   G2 phase
    D   S phase
    E   O phase

49. Which of the following statements describes genetic heterogeneity?

    A   It is a phenomenon in which genes interact with other factors in ways not well understood and difficult to quantify
    B   It means that a single gene can give rise to multiple phenotypes or disorders
    C   It means that different genotypes cause the same phenotype and are associated with the same risks of developing the phenotype or disorder
    D   It means that different genotypes cause the same phenotype but each genotype is associated with very different risks
    E   It means that multiple genes give rise to multiple phenotypes or disorders

50. Which of the following is associated with schizophrenia?

    A   45, X
    B   45, X/46, XX
    C   47, XYY
    D   Trisomy 16
    E   Trisomy 21

51. What is the prevalence rate of schizophrenia in 22q11.2 syndrome?

A   10%
B   25%
C   50%
D   65%
E   90%

52. What is the lifetime empirical risk of developing schizophrenia in offspring when both parents have schizophrenia?

A   6%
B   10%
C   13%
D   46%
E   56%

53. Which of the following chromosome pairs indicate genome-wide significant evidence for linkage for bipolar affective disorder types 1 and 2?

A   Chromosomes 10q and 12q
B   Chromosomes 2p and 4p
C   Chromosomes 2q and 4q
D   Chromosomes 6p and 8p
E   Chromosomes 6q and 8q

54. What is the most common comorbidity seen in a familial subtype of bipolar affective disorder?

A   Generalised anxiety disorder
B   Obsessive–compulsive disorder
C   Panic disorder
D   Phobic disorder
E   Somatoform disorder

55. Which allele is associated with the risk for major depression and suicidality in patients exposed to stressful life events?

A   Deletion allele
B   Insertion allele
C   Inversion allele
D   Recombinant allele
E   Translocation allele

56. Which of the following is consistent with comparative genomic use?

A   Macroarray analysis
B   Microarray analysis
C   Microformat analysis
D   Real-time, polymerase chain reaction gene, expression profiling
E   Microsatellite analysis

GENETICS: BEHAVIOURAL GENETICS

57. What is epistasis in behavioural genetics?

A   Gene–environment correlation
B   Gene–environment interaction

C   Non-additive interaction of alleles at different loci (gene–gene interaction)
D   Non-additive interaction of alleles within a locus
E   Responsible for the additive genetic variance

58. Which of the following observations is the best way to examine the effects of environmental sharing in twins?

A   Dizygotic twins reared in different environments
B   Dizygotic twins reared in the same environment
C   Monozygotic twins reared in different environments
D   Monozygotic twins reared in same environment
E   Twins who are mistaken about their zygosity

59. Which of the following statements about path analysis in qualitative genetics is correct?

A   It estimates genetic and environmental contributions using a simple diagrammatic method
B   It is a traditional twin design to represent genetic data for showing genetic and environmental contributions
C   It is a type of multiple regression analysis used in genetics
D   It is an eclectic mix of various appropriate statistical methods used in genetics
E   It is a representation of raw data that is then analysed according to the principles of 'model fitting' in genetics

60. The commonest cause of profound intellectual disability in girls and women is Rett's disorder. Which of the following statements about Rett's disorder is correct?

A   Approximately 99.5% of cases are a single occurrence in a family
B   Gene mutation occurs in the *MECP5* gene
C   It is an autosomal dominant condition
D   It is inherited as an X-linked recessive condition
E   There is no pervasive growth failure

61. Which of the following types of schizophrenia is less familial and also associated with a lower monozygotic twin concordance rate?

A   Catatonic schizophrenia
B   Hebephrenic schizophrenia
C   Paranoid schizophrenia
D   Residual schizophrenia
E   Simple schizophrenia

62. The heritability of social anxiety disorder is 25% in male twins. What is the heritability in female twins?

A   25%
B   40%
C   50%
D   65%
E   80%

63. Which of the following syndromes is caused by microdeletion of 7q 11?

A   Angelman's syndrome
B   Cri-du-chat syndrome
C   DiGeorge's syndrome
D   Prader–Willi syndrome
E   Williams' syndrome

64. Which of the following conditions is caused by CGG trinucleotide repeat?

A   Fragile X syndrome
B   Friedreich's ataxia
C   Huntington's disease
D   Myoclonic dystrophy
E   Myoclonus epilepsy

GENETICS: ENDOPHENOTYPES

65. P300 amplitude elicited from visual odd ball task is used as an endophenotype of alcohol dependence. What is a P300 amplitude reduction due to?

A   Craving
B   Executive dysfunction
C   Impulsivity
D   Sensation seeking
E   Tolerance

66. Who proposed the concept of endophenotypes in psychiatry?

A   Falconer
B   Gottesman and Shields
C   Gregor Mendel
D   John and Lewis
E   Michael Rutter

67. Which of the following statements about an endophenotype is most accurate?

A   Endophenotypes and the illness co-segregate
B   Endophenotypes are described in family members of affected individuals
C   Endophenotypes are not heritable
D   Endophenotypes are rarely seen in a normal population
E   Endophenotypes are state dependent

GENETICS: GENETIC EPIDEMIOLOGY

68. Collaborative studies on genetics of alcoholism study have found some chromosomes and genes that are involved in alcohol dependence. Which of the following is associated with alcohol dependence?

A $5HTT$ gene
B   Chromosomes 14 and 22
C $DAT1$ gene
D $GABAb$ gene
E $GABRA2$ gene

GENETICS: GENE–ENVIRONMENT INTERACTION

69. Which of the following statements about familiality and genetic factors in schizophrenia is correct?

A   Common high penetrance variants are high-risk factors for schizophrenia

B   Common variants in the genes neuregulin-1 and dysbindin and D-amino acid oxidase activator contribute a small increase to the risk for schizophrenia

C   Dizygotic co-twins are 50% concordant for the disorder

D   Monozygotic co-twins are 95% concordant for the disorder

E   Multiple low-penetrance common variants contribute little or no risk for schizophrenia

70. You analysed twin studies in a rare psychiatric disorder. The concordance rate of development of the disorder in both monozygotic and dizygotic twins was 30%. What does this mean?

A   Environmental factors play a more important role in the development of disorder than genetic factors

B   Genetic factors play a more important role in the development of disorder than the environment

C   There is no role for environmental factors in the development of the disorder

D   There is no role for genetic factors in the development of the disorder

E   This finding does not give any conclusive evidence as to whether genetic or environmental factors play a major role in the development of the disorder

71. In which of the following conditions is linkage analysis useful?

A   Autism

B   Bipolar affective disorder

C   Depression

D   Huntington's disease

E   Schizophrenia

72. In which of the following situations is heritability of a mental disorder noticed to be increased?

A   Having a secure job

B   Living in urban areas

C   Married status

D   No financial worries

E   Religious upbringing

73. In a gene–environment interaction, what do structured situations mean?

A   How society structures the environment

B   Situations that provide relatively unambiguous cues to guide behaviour

C   Situations in which individuals' genetic make-up structures the environment

D   Situations in which individuals can structure the environment

E   Situations in which researchers structure the environment

EPIDEMIOLOGY: SURVEYS ACROSS THE LIFESPAN

74. What is the prevalence of specific phobias in patients with learning disability?

A   1.5%

B   2.5%

C   3%

D   6%

E   7%

75. Which of the following factors is associated with an increased risk of suicide in patients with schizophrenia?

A   Good compliance with treatment

B   High education level

C   Low IQ
D   Low aggression
E   Poor insight

76. Which of the following increases the risk of suicide in patients with schizophrenia?

A   Delusions
B   Depression
C   Hallucinations
D   Negative symptoms
E   Thought disorders

77. Which of the following factors is associated with the highest risk of suicide in patients with schizophrenia?

A   African–Caribbean ethnicity
B   Being a female
C   Delayed discharge from hospital
D   First episode in later years of life
E   White ethnicity

78. Which country has a higher female than male suicide rate?

A   China
B   Denmark
C   India
D   New Zealand
E   Switzerland

79. Which of the following statements about the prevalence of schizophrenia is correct?

A   Developing countries have a higher prevalence
B   Life-time prevalence is 4/1000
C   Migrants have a lower risk
D   There are significant differences between male and female prevalence
E   There are significant differences in urban and rural prevalence

80. The study of the aetiology and ethnicity of schizophrenia and other psychoses investigated the clinical and social determinants of duration of untreated psychosis (DUP) in patients with a first episode of psychosis. Which of the following was associated with a longer DUP?

A   Affective psychosis
B   Employment
C   Frank psychotic symptoms
D   Help-seeking behaviour of family
E   Insidious onset

81. Approximately what percentage of patients with schizophrenia is implicated in homicides in the UK?

A   0.5%
B   0.8%
C   1%
D   3%
E   5%

82. How common are psychotic symptoms in patients with delirium?

A   25%
B   50%

C   70%
D   80%
E   100%

83. Which of the following increases the incidence of schizophrenia?

A   Abnormal motor and speech development before 2 years
B   Being born in developing countries
C   Being born in developed countries
D   Left-handedness
E   Right-handedness

84. What is the best short-term predictor of relapse in a patient with psychosis?

A   Duration of untreated psychosis
B   Heavy cannabis use
C   Highly expressed emotions
D   Stressful life event
E   Withdrawal of antipsychotics

85. Which part of the UK has the lowest suicide rate for men?

A   East of England
B   East Midlands
C   North west
D   North east
E   West Midlands

86. What percentage of people with mental illness consumes tobacco regularly in the UK?

A   30%
B   40%
C   50%
D   60%
E   70%

87. What is the estimated rate of suicide in the world?

A   1 every 10 seconds
B   1 every 20 seconds
C   1 every 30 seconds
D   1 every 40 seconds
E   1 every 50 seconds

88. Which of the following is a self-rating scale?

A   Brief psychiatric rating scale
B   General health questionnaire
C   Hamilton's rating scale for depression
D   Montgomery–Asberg depression rating scale
E   Yale–Brown obsessive compulsive scale

89. Which of the following is a measure of disease frequency?

A   Absolute risk reduction
B   Attributable risk
C   Incidence
D   Number needed to treat
E   Odds ratio

90. Which of the following rating scales is most sensitive to change in depressive symptoms?

    A   Beck's depression inventory
    B   Bech–Rafaelsen melancholia scale
    C   Hamilton rating scale for depression
    D   Major depression inventory
    E   Montgomery–Asberg depression rating scale

91. Which of the following is used to investigate heterogeneity?

    A   Cox's proportional hazard analysis
    B   Fixed effect analysis
    C   Galbraith's plot
    D   Kaplan–Meier method
    E   Log-rank test

92. A study was designed to investigate both mania and depression. Which of the following scales will be the most appropriate?

    A   Bech–Rafaelsen rating scale
    B   Beck's depression inventory
    C   Hopelessness scale
    D   Young's mania rating scale
    E   Zung self-rating scale

93. Which of the following is a personality assessment scale based on an individual's coping strategies?

    A   Defensive functioning scale
    B   Global assessment of relational functioning
    C   Million clinical mini-inventory
    D   Minnesota multiphasic personality inventory
    E   Rorschach's test

ADVANCED PSYCHOLOGICAL PROCESSES AND TREATMENTS: NEUROPSYCHOLOGY

94. Which of the following is thought to be the defining feature of an amnestic syndrome?

    A   Intact iconic memory
    B   Intact procedural memory
    C   Intact semantic memory
    D   Loss of immediate memory
    E   Retained anterograde memory

95. Which of the following neuropsychological abnormalities is found in patients with schizophrenia?

    A   Astereognosis
    B   Impairments in executive functioning
    C   Impairments in intelligence
    D   Impairments in long-term memory
    E   Impairments in procedural memory

ADVANCED PSYCHOLOGICAL PROCESSES AND TREATMENTS: PERSONALITY AND PERSONALITY DISORDER

96. In the early twentieth century, Sheldon tried to establish a link between body type and personality. Which of the following traits relates to food, comfort, people and affection?

    A   Cerebrotonic
    B   Ectomorphic
    C   Mesomorphic
    D   Somatotonic
    E   Viscerotonic

97. Which of the following is included in the general diagnostic guidelines for personality disorders?

    A   Attributable to other psychiatric disorder
    B   Distress to others but not to oneself
    C   Harmonious attitudes and behaviours
    D   Maladaptive behaviour
    E   Periodic presentation

98. Which of the following is included in the diagnostic criteria of the ICD-10 diagnosis of dissocial personality disorder?

    A   Blames self
    B   Conduct disorder in childhood
    C   Increased interest in sexual experiences
    D   Irresponsible attitude
    E   Persistent irritability

99. According to thepsychodynamic theory of aetiology of personality disorders, difficulties in the oedipal phase of psychosexual development are implicated. In which of the following personality disorders might this be the case?

    A   Anxious–avoidant personality disorder
    B   Dependant personality disorder
    C   Emotionally unstable, dissocial personality disorder
    D   Histrionic personality disorder
    E   Obsessive–compulsive personality disorder

100. With regard to dialectic behaviour therapy (DBT) and suicidality in borderline personality disorder, which of the following statements is correct?

    A   It is associated with higher medical risk if suicide was attempted
    B   DBT appears to result in reduced suicide attempts
    C   Effectiveness of DBT is attributed to general factors associated with expert psychotherapy
    D   Patients receiving DBT are twice as likely to make a suicide attempt
    E   Patients receiving DBT are more likely to require hospitalisation due to suicidal ideations

ADVANCED PSYCHOLOGICAL PROCESSES AND TREATMENTS: DEVELOPMENTAL PSYCHOPATHOLOGY (INCLUDING TEMPERAMENT)

101. Which of the following statements is most accurate about the strange situation experiment?

- A   Almost a third of children have anxious avoidant attachment styles
- B   Almost three-quarters of children are found to be securely attached
- C   It was devised by Ainsworth and Wittig in 1869
- D   Four types of attachment behaviours were identified from the experiment
- E   The baby treats the stranger and the mother in the same way in the anxious–resistant type of attachment

102. Which of the following statements about Piaget's four stages of development is correct?

- A   Concrete operational stage occurs between age 2 and 7 years
- B   Egocentrism happens in the formal operational stage
- C   Idea manipulations and propositions happen in the formal operational stage
- D   Object permanence develops in the preoperational stage
- E   Transductive reasoning develops in the concrete operational stage

103. Which of the following statements about Freud's stages of psychosexual development is correct?

- A   Balance of id, ego and superego is best maintained in the genital stage
- B   Latency period spans 3–6 years
- C   Oedipus complex develops in the latency phase
- D   Parents are seen as authority figures in the phallic stage
- E   Powerful demands in the form of heterosexual desires occur in the genital stage

104. Which of the following is the most accurate statement about Kohlberg's theory of moral development?

- A   Conventional morality is seen after the age of 5 years
- B   Kohlberg differentiated two types of moral orientation: heteronomous and autonomous
- C   Postconventional morality includes interpersonal concordance orientation
- D   Preconventional morality corresponds to a preoperational stage in Piaget's development
- E   Universal ethical principle is stage 5 of moral development

105. Which of the following is the stage in development of gender identity as suggested by Kohlberg?

- A   Gender comparison
- B   Gender consistency
- C   Gender instability
- D   Gender questioning
- E   Gender relativism

ADVANCED PSYCHOLOGICAL PROCESSES AND TREATMENTS: THERAPY MODELS, METHODS, PROCESSES AND OUTCOMES

106. Which of the following statements about psychodynamic interpersonal therapy is correct?

- A   It was developed by Linehan
- B   It has five components

C   It is suitable only for a short-term intervention
D   There is no evidence base to support its use
E   It was originally called 'the conversational model'

107. According to cognitive–analytic therapy, which of the following statements about the procedural sequence model is correct?

A   Faulty procedures include snags, traps and dilemmas
B   It involves only feelings and acting-out behaviour
C   It is based on Sigmund Freud's principles of human psychosexual development
D   It is of a limited value in depressed patients
E   It was developed to understand acting-out behaviour

108. Which of the following statements about motivational interviewing is correct?

A   One of the techniques is to emphasise personal choice and control
B   It is useful only to manage alcohol addiction
C   Strategies include setting tasks such as activity scheduling
D   The patient's family are the focus of the therapy
E   This approach was developed to assess at which stage of change the patient is

109. Which of the following statements about behaviour therapy is correct?

A   Behaviour therapy is based on operant conditioning
B   Behaviour modification is based on classic conditioning
C   Flooding has been found to be minimally useful for the treatment of phobias
D   Reciprocal inhibition occurs in aversion therapy
E   Systematic desensitisation represents a form of counter-conditioning

110. Four stages of treatment are described in DBT for patients with borderline personality disorder. Which of the following statements is correct?

A   Stage 1 involves emotionally processing the past
B   Stage 2 involves achieving behavioural control
C   Stage 3 refers to the capacity to experience sustained joy
D   Stage 4 refers to resolving problems in living
E   The last two stages are unlikely to be available in most public healthcare settings

111. A 15-year-old boy was caught shoplifting. He was known to play truant and lie frequently. There were some concerns about him because he had been more aggressive and getting into fights with the children in the neighbourhood. Which intervention is recommended to manage his presentation?

A   Cognitive–behavioural therapy
B   DBT
C   Habit reversal and competing interests
D   Multisystemic therapy
E   Positive reinforcement and punishment

112. Which of the following is a behavioural technique that increases a desired behaviour?

A   Extinction
B   Stimulus control
C   Shaping
D   Time out
E   Diaries

113. A 24-year-old solider who returned from Afghanistan presented with recurrent flashbacks and nightmares. Which of the following is the psychological therapy of choice?

A   Cognitive–analytic therapy
B   DBT
C   Eye movement desensitisation and reprocessing
D   Interpersonal psychotherapy
E   Systemic family therapy

114. Which of the following statements about Freud's psychoanalytic theory is correct?

A   Ego is the moral judicial part of the personality
B   Ego is the presocialised part of the personality
C   Moral conflicts happen between the super-ego and the ego
D   Reality principle is associated with the super-ego
E   Super-ego deals with deferred gratification

115. Which of the following statements about psychological interventions in patients with borderline personality disorder is correct?

A   Art therapy is an effective treatment for these patients
B   Cognitive–behaviour therapy (CBT) delivered to patients focuses on the 'here and now'
C   Complementary therapies have gradually gained popularity in the management of these patients
D   Number of sessions of CBT offered to patients is significantly less than for those with axis I disorders
E   Systems training for emotional predictability and problem solving is a CBT-based skills development package

116. Which of the following statements about systems training for emotional predictability and problem solving is correct?

A   Family and significant others are part of each session delivered
B   It is delivered over 20 weeks
C   The sessions of the therapy last 50–60 minutes
D   It uses a psychodynamic approach
E   It is used primarily for patients with depression

117. Which of the following terms is used in the description of thought processes in cognitive–analytical therapy?

A   Altruism
B   Black-and-white thinking
C   Minimisation
D   Projective identification
E   Snags

118. Which of the following statements about psychological therapies for a bipolar affective disorder (BPAD) is correct?

A   Aims of psychological therapy include reduction in mood fluctuations and maintaining a stable mental state
B   CBT is commonly used in children with bipolar affective disorder
C   Individually structured therapy is best used in the acute phase of the disorder
D   There is a good evidence base for psychological therapy to increase medication adherence
E   There is a good evidence base for psychological therapies in managing comorbid substance misuse in a BPAD

119. Which of the following statements about family-based psychological interventions for adolescents with anorexia is correct?

    A   Family interventions should focus on how the disorder impacts on family relationships
    B   Issues such as consent should be overridden by parents or clinicians
    C   Seeing patients and parents separately is not beneficial; they should be seen together
    D   There is a large evidence base for its efficacy in anorexia nervosa
    E   Therapist should not allow parents to take a central role in the early stages of treatment

120. With regard to CBT and psychosis, which of the following psychotic symptoms has shown better outcomes for CBT?

    A   Audible thoughts
    B   Delusional beliefs
    C   Delusional memory
    D   Misidentification
    E   Visual hallucinations

121. Which of the following is a cognitive bias in Beck's theory of depression?

    A   Arbitrary inference
    B   Over-projection
    C   Projection bias
    D   Selective cognition
    E   Selective exaggeration

122. Which of the following is considered a high-intensity psychological treatment?

    A   CBT
    B   Computerised CBT
    C   Guided self-help
    D   Non-facilitated self-help
    E   Psychoeducational groups

ADVANCED PSYCHOLOGICAL PROCESSES AND TREATMENTS: PSYCHOSOCIAL INFLUENCES

123. Which of the following statements about the social readjustment rating scale (SRRS) is correct?

    A   SRRS was generated from the work of Lazarus
    B   SRRS assumes that any change in life is by definition stressful
    C   There are 40 life events included in the SRRS
    D   Total score of life change unit (LCU) > 200 in a year is classed as a major crisis
    E   Total score of LCU < 200 in a year is not classed as a crisis

Answers: MCQs

1. B Hemiballismus

This rare movement disorder occurs after a lesion in subthalamic nucleus, resulting in involuntary movements of the extremities on the side of the body. There is involvement of either proximal and/or distal extremities and occasionally the face.

Table 2.1 Movement disorders and affected areas of brain	
Movement disorder	**Lesion in brain**
Bradykinesia	Striatal over-activity due to lack of dopaminergic inhibition
Hemiballismus	Subthalamic nucleus lesion
Parkinson's disease	Substantia nigra–depigmentation, loss of dopamine neurons, presence of Lewy bodies
	Also affected–locus ceruleus, nucleus basalis, raphe and ventral tegmental area
Huntington's disease	Degeneration of striatum (mainly caudate nucleus)
Wilson's disease	Copper deposition in lenticular nuclei (pallidus and putamen)
	Abnormalities also found in the caudate, thalamus, cerebellar nuclei and white matter

2. B Golgi cells

Cellular components of the cerebellum include neurons and axons. Golgi cells are the smallest and Purkinje cells are the largest of all neurons in the cerebellum. There are five types of cells found in the cerebellum, forming three distinct layers:

>   Molecular layer (superficial layer) – stellate and basket cells
>   Purkinje layer (middle layer) –Purkinje cells
>   Granular layer (deepest layer) – granular and Golgi cells.

Granular cells are the only excitatory cells, whereas stellate, Golgi, Purkinje and basket cells are inhibitory cells in the cerebellum.

3. C Lateral fissure separates the temporal and frontal lobes

The cerebral cortex is the outermost neural tissue covering the cerebrum and cerebellum, dividing it into the left and right hemispheres. It is folded into deep groves known as sulci.

Table 2.2 Division of the cerebral cortex

Structure	Subdivision
Lateral fissure (also called sylvian fissure)	Temporal and frontal lobes
Central sulcus (also called rolandic fissure)	Frontal and parietal lobes
Parieto-occipital sulcus	Occipital and parietal lobes on the medial surface only
No clear boundary structure	Occipital and parietal lobes on the lateral surface
Longitudinal (also called sagittal) fissure	Cerebrum into right and left hemisphere

4. D Optic nerve

Cranial nerves with sensory component only–three nerves: olfactory, optic and vestibulocochlear nerves (I, II and IX).

Cranial nerves with motor component only–Five nerves: oculomotor, trochlear, abducens, accessory and hypoglossal nerves (III, IV, VI, XI and XII).

In addition, the following four cranial nerves also have an autonomic component–oculomotor, facial, glossopharyngeal and vagus nerves (III, VII, IX and X).

Mnemonic to remember which cranial nerves are sensory (S), motor (M) or both (B) in order of sequence from I to XII:

Some **s**ay **m**oney **m**atters **b**ut **m**y **b**rother **s**ays **b**ig **b**rains **m**atter **m**ost.

5. E Trapezoid body

The other options are correct for the visual pathway.

Heschl's gyrus is the auditory cortex.

Table 2.3 Visual and auditory pathways

Visual pathway	Auditory pathway
Myer's loop, lateral geniculate body, tectum	Medial geniculate body, inferior colliculus, lateral lemniscus, trapezoid body, superior olivary complex
Other structures that are easy to identify in options: corner, lens, retina, optic nerve, optic chiasma, optic tract, optic radiation, visual cortex	Other structures that are easily identified: cochlea, cochlear nerve, cochlear nucleus

Morgan G, Butler S. Seminars in Basic Neuroscience. London: Gaskell, 1998: 16–20.

6. A Changes in locus ceruleus

In Parkinson's disease, there is depigmentation of the locus ceruleus and substantia nigra, particularly the zona compacta. The macroscopic changes in Huntington's disease are a small brain with reduced mass, dilatation of the lateral and third ventricle, marked atrophy of the cerebral cortex, particularly the frontal lobe gyri, and marked atrophy of the corpus striatum, particularly the caudate lobe.

7. C Hirano's bodies in hippocampus

Microscopic changes seen in Alzheimer's disease:

- Diffuse neuronal loss is a prominent feature of late stage Alzheimer's disease. Neocortex frequently shows astrocytosis and activated microglia.
- Hirano's bodies are neuronal inclusions and best seen in the hippocampus.
- There is a loss of cholinergic neurons, particularly in the temporal cortex and nucleus of Meynert in the basal forebrain. There is also loss of adrenergic neurons in the locus ceruleus in the brain stem. However, most important are the amyloid plaques and neurofibrillary tangles. Ballooned neurons (Pick's cells) and Pick's bodies are found in Pick's disease. In addition, Hirano bodies can also be found, although fewer than in Alzheimer's disease.

8. E Neurilemmomas

Gliomas are derived from glial cells and their precursors. These tumours incude astrocytomas, oligodendrocytomas and ependymomas. The cerebral tumour that has the maximum frequency of occurrence is a glioma. The following cerebral tumours are arranged in relative frequency of occurrence: gliomas, metastases, meningeal tumours, pituitary adenomas, neurilemmomas, haemangioblastomas and medulloblastomas.

Neurilemmomas are also known as schwannomas. They are derived from Schwann cells and also include acoustic neuromas.

9. D Neurofibrillary tangles are intraneuronal aggregations

Amyloid plaques are extracellular, insoluble, fibrillary and non-fibrillary material composed of BA4 amyloid protein. Deposits are of several types, the main ones being neuritic and dense plaques.

Neurofibrillary tangles are intraneuronal aggregations of insoluble tau protein. Six isoforms of normal tau are known. Hyperphosphorylation of all these six isoforms is characteristic of Alzheimer's disease. Most of the tangles appear in the hippocampus first.

Both are not pathognomonic for Alzheimer's dementia because they are seen in other conditions.

Amyloid plaques are also seen in Down's syndrome and amyloid angiopathy.

Neurofibrillary tangles are also seen in Down's syndrome, dementia pugilistica, progressive supranuclear palsy, frontotemporal dementia with parkinsonism (FTDP-17) and Hallervorden–Spatz disease (progressive extrapyramidal dysfunction and dementia).

10. A Amyloid plaques

Bielschowsky's staining is a silver stain used to demonstrate amyloid plaques and neurofibrillary tangles in Alzheimer's disease. Other silver methods used are: Gallyas and Bodian stains, thioflavine stain and Congo red. These lesions can also be demonstrated by immunohistochemistry techniques. Do remember that the haematoxylin and eosin stain can also be used although it does not demonstrate the full burden of deposits and tangles.

11. B NREM stage 2

The percentage of sleep time in young adult non-rapid eye movement (NREM) stage 1 is 5%, stage 2 is 45%, stages 3 and 4 is 25%, and REM is 25%. The percentage of stage 3, 4 and REM decreases with age. Stage 1 is the lightest stage of sleep which is characterised by peacefulness, episodic body movements, and low pulse rate, respiration and blood pressure. Stage 2 has the largest percentage of the sleep time. Stages 3 and 4 are the deepest, most relaxed stage of the sleep. In this stage sleep walking and bed wetting may occur. In the REM stage, there would be dreaming and an absence of skeletal muscle movement. A person may have penile or clitoris erection, increased pulse, respiration and blood pressure.

12. D 13 μm

Aα, Aβ, Aγ, Aδ, B and C afferents have a diameter of 15, 8, 5, 13, 3 and 1 μm, respectively.

Aα is a muscle spindle afferent and Aβ carries cutaneous touch and pressure sensation.

Aγ has cutaneous temperature and pain afferents and B nerves have sympathetic preganglionic neurons. The pain/temperature afferents are sympathetic postganglion neurons.

13. C 8–13 Hz

α Waves are the dominant posterior rhythm and present when an individual is awake but with the eyes closed. When the individual opens his or her eyes, the α rhythm is replaced by random activity.

Table 2.4 Electroencephalogram		
Waveform	**Frequency (Hz)**	**Seen in the following condition**
δ	<4	Normal in sleep
θ	4–8	It can be present in 15% people under normal conditions
α	8–13	Disappear when eyes are opened
		Prominent in occipital area
β	>13	Can be seen with eyes open or closed
		Barbiturates, alcohol, benzodiazepines and anxiety can increase activity

14. E Triphasic 1–2 Hz discharge

The following conditions are matched with appropriate electroencephalogram (EEG) changes seen on investigation:

Absent seizure – 3-Hz spike-and-wave activity
Infantile spasm – hypsarrhythmia
Variant Creutzfeldt–Jakob disease–normal or non-specific EEG
Herpes simplex encephalitis–periodic discharge with focal δ activity over temporal lobes
Sporadic Creutzfeldt–Jakob disease – Triphasic 1–2 Hz discharge.

15. B Acetylcholine nicotinic

Ionotropic receptor for neurotransmitter includes glutamate, AMPA-K, γ-aminobutyric acid A (GABA-A), acetylcholine, nicotinic and glycine, serotonin (5-hydroxytryptamine [5-HT$_3$]) and purines. The metabotropic receptors are activated by glutamate (or mGluR), GABA-B, acetylcholine muscarinic, dopamine D$_1$/D$_2$-receptors, serotonin 5-HT$_1$-/5-HT$_2$-receptors, noradrenaline, histamine H$_1$-/H$_2$-/H$_3$-receptors, all types of neuropeptides and adenosine.

16. C Down-regulation of glucocorticoid receptor

The following changes are seen in patients with depression and other mood disorders:

Hypersecretion of corticotrophin-releasing hormone and adrenal vasopressin
Hypercortisolaemia in serum, urine, cerebrospinal fluid and saliva
Enlarged hypothalamus, and pituitary and adrenal glands
Exaggerated cortisol response to ACTH (adrenocorticotrophic hormone).

17. A Cholecystokinin

Dopamine, noradrenaline, adrenaline, serotonin, acetylcholine and histamine are the monoamine receptors. GABA, glycine and glutamate are the amino acid receptors. Endorphins, cholecystokinin, angiotensin II, neurotensin and corticotrophin-releasing hormone are peptide neurotransmitters.

18. E Serotonin

As far as precursors are concerned, choline and acetyl-coenzyme A are precursors of acetylcholine. L-Tyrosine, L-dopa and dopamine are precursors of noradrenaline. L-Tryptophan is the precursor of serotonin. L-Tyrosine and L-dopa are precursors of dopamine and histidine is the precursor of histamine.

19. A Decreased glutamatergic function at NMDA

There is growing evidence that glutamate and schizophrenia are related. Glutamate has three types of receptors: NMDA, AMPA and kainate. Psychotic symptoms can be produced by the decreased glutamatergic function of NMDA, and increased function at AMPA and kainate receptors. Recent research is looking at developing drugs that work at the glycine site of NMDA receptors which can help in treating some psychotic symptoms in schizophrenia.

20. E Histidine

As far as precursors are concerned, choline and acetyl-coenzyme A are precursors of acetylcholine. L-tyrosine, L-dopa and dopamine are precursors of noradrenaline. L-Tryptophan is the precursor of serotonin. L-Tyrosine and L-dopa are precursors of dopamine and histidine is the precursor of histamine.

21. E Reduced medial temporal lobe width at the level of the brain stem

MRI: MRI studies confirm the finding of postmortem studies that the disease process in Alzheimer's disease starts in and around the hippocampus. In the earlier stages, there is progressive atrophy in the medical temporal lobe and temporoparietal cortex. In the later stages, the frontal lobes are affected as well. The rate of generalised atrophy progression is >5% per year. In addition, there is a moderate increase in deep white matter lesions.

CT scan: the Oxford project to investigate memory and ageing found that there is marked reduction in medial temporal lobe thickness at the level of the brain stem in confirmed cases of Alzheimer's dementia. Initial CT studies also found that there is a 10-fold increase in a rate of ventricular dilatation, by 15% each year.

22. A Anatomical structures

The main types of MRI sequences and its advantages:

T1-weighted image – high resolution and definition of anatomical structures
T2 weighted image – high contrast and definition of soft tissue
Proton density-weighted image – high brain/cerebrospinal fluid contrast.

T2-weighted and proton density images are good for identifying white matter lesions and smaller infarcts. In addition, these images are sensitive to changes in water content. Cerebrospinal fluid appears dark on T1 and proton density images, whereas it appears bright on T2-weighted images. On imaging, a combination of sequences is used for the best images of anatomy and pathology.

23. B [^{11}C]Raclopride

[^{11}C]-Hyoscine: muscarinic receptors

[^{18}F]-Flumazenil: benzodiazepine receptors

[^{18}F]-Flurodopa: presynaptic dopamine synthesis

[^{18}F]Setoperone and [^{11}C]-ketanserin: 5-hydroxytryptophan 2 receptors

24. E Stands for single photon emission computed tomography

This uses manufactured radioactive compound to study the regional differences in the cerebral blood flow within the brain area. It is a high-resolution imaging technique that is used to record the pattern of photon emission from the bloodstream. It is based on the level of perfusion in different areas of brain.

25. C 0.3–2.0 T

MRI entered into clinical practice in 1982. It has become the test of choice for psychiatrists and neurologists. It does not involve the absorption of the X-rays; rather it involves nuclear magnetic resonance. MRI scanners collect the emissions of individual nuclei and then two-dimensional pictures are generated using computer analysis. The unit used for MRI magnets is the tesla (T). It is used for magnetic field strength. In clinical practice, MRI uses magnets that are in range 0.3–2.0 T.

26. B 3 mg

The usual range of paliperidone is 3–12 mg daily. In cases of renal impairment, when estimated glomerular filtration rate (eGFR) is 50–80 mL/min per 1.73 m^2 then maximum *British National Formulary* (BNF) dose is 6 mg. If the eGFR is 10–50 mL/min per 1.73 m^2 then the maximum BNF dose is 3 mg/day. If the eGFR is <10 mL/min per 1.73 m^2 it has to be avoided. Paliperidone injection is indicated for maintenance treatment of patients with schizophrenia who had responded to risperidone or paliperidone tablets.

27. B Haloperidol

In general, caution should be exercised in using those drugs that are mainly hepatically metabolised when dealing with patients with liver impairment. Amisulpiride and paliperidone are mainly excreted unchanged through the kidneys. Most other antipsychotics, including haloperidol, are metabolised in the liver. However, haloperidol is recommended as the drug of choice in clinical practice because of a good evidence base.

28. A Antagonist of glutamate receptor

Acamprosate is a taurine analogue that appears to act centrally on glutamate and γ-aminobutyric acid. The mechanism of action is not known. It is initiated after abstinence has been achieved and it should be maintained if the person relapses in alcohol drinking. It has a modest treatment effect.

29. E Sodium valproate

Benzodiazepine and barbiturates enhance the hyperpolarisation effect of γ-aminobutyric acid (GABA) on glutamate neurons. Carbamazepine and phenytoin reduce high-frequency repetitive firing by blocking glutamate ionotropic receptors, and make their ion channels less permeable to sodium and calcium. Sodium valproate blocks the transaminase enzyme that converts GABA to glutamate which in turn increases the GABA's time in synaptic cleft.

30. D Oxazepam

Table 2.5 Commonly used benzodiazepines and their half-lives

Drug	Half-life (hours)	Effects of increasing age
Clobazam	12–60	Elimination half-life decreased
Diazepam	20–90	Elimination half-life increased
Flurazepam	40–100	Toxicity increased
Alprazolam	6–20	Elimination half-life decreased
Flunitrazepam	20–30	Little effect
Lorazepam	10–20	Little effect
Nitrazepam	20–30	Elimination half-life increased
Oxazepam	4–14	No effect
Temazepam	8–22	Little effect
Triazolam	5–10	Elimination half-life increased
Chlordiazepoxide	5–30	Elimination half-life increased

31. B Aripiprazole

Partial agonists bind and activate a given receptor, but have only partial efficacy at the receptor relative to a full agonist. Amisulpiride is primarily a D_2- and D_3-receptor antagonist. Aripiprazole is a partial D_2-receptor agonist. Ziprasidone blocks D_2-, D_3- and 5-HT$_{1D}$-receptors and stimulates 5HT$_{1A}$-receptors. Paliperidone is a metabolite of risperidone and blocks D_2- and 5-HT$_{2A}$-receptors. Clobazam is a γ-aminobutyric acid agonist.

32. D It is also available as a depot injection formulation

Paliperidone is available as a depot formulation (as paliperidone palmitate) in addition to aboral formulation. It is a metabolite (not a precursor) of risperidone and is licensed for use in schizophrenia where there is response to risperidone or oral paliperidone, but not in bipolar disorder. It blocks D_2- and 5-HT-receptors including α_1-, α_2-adrenergic receptors and H_1 histamine receptors.

33. C St John's wort

St John's wort reduces the anticoagulant effect of warfarin and increases the risk of thrombosis. All other drugs mentioned in the question increase its anticoagulant effect. St John's wort is an inducer of intestinal and hepatic cytochromes CYP450-P3A4 and CYP450-P2C. It significantly reduces plasma concentrations of digoxin and indinavir (a drug used in the treatment of HIV). According to a number of case reports, St John's wort has lowered the plasma concentrations of theophylline, ciclosporin, warfarin, gliclazide, atorvastatin and the combined oral contraceptive pill, and has led to treatment failure (BNF).

34. C St John's wort

It is an inducer of intestinal and hepatic cytochromes CYP450-P3A4 and CYP450-P2C. St John's wort reduces the contraceptive effects of oestrogen. Other drugs mentioned in the question do not interact with contraceptive pills. Fluoxetine is a strong enzyme inhibitor and so inhibits metabolism of various drugs that are metabolised by the cytochrome system. Venlafaxine also inhibits metabolism of various drugs. Valproate has a variable interaction with various drugs because it can reduce as well as enhance metabolism.

35. C Lofepramine

The main difference between the various preparations of antidepressants is the side-effect profile. Lofepramine does not contribute to weight gain but all tricyclic antidepressants are associated with more risks because of the risk of overdose.

36. E Olanzapine embonate

Intramuscular olanzapine has a safety profile similar to oral olanzapine with the exception that it can cause post-injection syndrome in a small proportion of patients (0.07–0.14%) . The symptoms and signs are similar to those of olanzapine overdose. It can start within an hour of injection and present with excessive sedation, agitation and/or a delirium-like picture. Complete recovery can be seen in 1–3 days after the injection.

37. C Impaired deglutition

Clozapine blocks M_1-, M_2-, M_3- and M_5-receptors whereas it stimulates M_4-receptors. Both M_3 and M_4-receptors are expressed in the salivary glands and have the opposite action with M_3-receptor blockade and M_4-receptor stimulation, both promoting hypersalivation. Clozapine also disturbs the swallowing of saliva. α_2-Receptor antagonism is also thought to be a contributing factor. This is not an extrapyramidal side effect.

38. C 150 mg/kg

In adult/child acetylcysteine is given by intravenous infusion, initially 150 mg/kg (maximum 16.5 g) over 15 minutes, then 50 mg/kg (maximum 5.5 g) over 4 hours than 100 mg/kg (maximum 11 g) over 16 hours.

A total dose of as little as 10–15 g (20–30 tablets) or 150 mg/kg of paracetamol ingested within 24 hours in one attempt or repeated attempts may cause severe hepatocellular necrosis and, much less frequently, renal tubular necrosis. Patients who have liver damage or are taking enzyme-inducing drugs may develop liver toxicity with as little as 75 mg/kg of paracetamol taken within 24 hours. The nausea and vomiting are the only early features of poisoning that usually settle within 24 hours. If the symptom persists and if it is associated with the onset of right subcostal pain and tenderness, this usually indicates development of hepatic necrosis. The liver damage is at its maximum 3–4 days after ingestion. The paracetamol overdose patient should be transferred to hospital urgently despite a lack of significant early symptoms. The activated charcoal administration should be considered if paracetamol were ingested within the previous hour and taken in excess of 150 mg/kg or 12 g, or in excess of 75 mg/kg for high-risk patients.

39. C Females are at lesser risk than males

The risk factors for neuroleptic malignant syndrome are male gender, high-potency antipsychotics (e.g. haloperidol), long-acting antipsychotics (e.g. depots), rapid increase or decrease in the dose of antipsychotics, and parenteral route of administration. There is some evidence for a family history posing a greater risk. It is not dose dependent and is more likely to occur in the early course of treatment. A low threshold of suspicion is important, particularly in the presence of several risk factors, to avoid missing this potentially life-threatening condition, which can be confused with other medical conditions such as catatonia, malignant hyperthermia, serotonin syndrome or infective illnesses such as encephalitis.

40. A Duloxetine

Tricyclic antidepressants, citalopram, escitalopram, paroxetine, sertraline, reboxetine and mirtazapine could be cross-tapered while switching to venlafaxine. On the other hand, it is advisable to withdraw fluoxetine, duloxetine and monoamine oxidase inhibitors and then start venlafaxine.

41. D 450 mg

Most studies suggest that the threshold for response is in the plasma level range of 350–420 µg/L. The plasma level varies according to gender and smoking status. The approximate dose for a male non-smoker is 350 mg/day and it is 550 mg/day for a male who has a smoking habit. Similarly for a female the approximate dose is 250 mg/day for a non-smoker and 450 mg/day for a smoker.

42. D 433 mg

Sodium valproate 500 mg is equivalent to 433 mg of valproic acid. Valproic acid 500 mg is equivalent to 538.2 mg semi-sodium valproate. Semi-sodium valproate, also called Depakote, is a combination of sodium valproate and valproic acid. Sodium valproate is also known as Epilim.

43. D Sertraline

Selective serotonin reuptake inhibitors are generally recommended post-myocardial infarction (MI). Mirtazepine is a suitable alternative. Sertraline is the preferred antidepressant after an MI and in heart failure. Caution is advised with the use of fluoxetine and paroxetine after an MI, although they are not contraindicated. Tricyclic antidepressants should be avoided after an MI because of their cardiotoxic potential. There is not enough evidence for the use of venlafaxine in this situation.

44. E Topiramate

It is reported to reduce drinking days and increases abstinence in an alcohol-dependent person. The exact mechanism of action is not known. It has antiepileptic and antimigraine action. It works by blocking voltage-sensitive sodium channels, inhibiting the release of glutamate; this potentiates the activity of γ-aminobutyric acid receptors, by inhibiting the carbonic anhydrase enzyme. The carbonic anhydrase inhibition may give rise to kidney stones and paraesthesia.

45. C 10 mg

Table 2.6 Diazepam equivalents	
Name	Dose (mg)
Chlordiazepoxide	25
Clonazepam	1–2
Diazepam	10
Lorazepam	1
Lormetazepam	1
Nitrazepam	10
Oxazepam	30
Temazepam	20

46. B Replication

This is a process of producing of new copies of DNA from template DNA which occurs during mitosis. Perfect duplication of DNA occurs due to error-checking and error-correcting mechanisms. Transcription is the synthesis of RNA from DNA. Translation is the process of producing proteins from RNA and consists of three steps: initiation, elongation and termination. Modification is a change in phenotype of an organism, which is caused by environmental changes and is not inheritable. Synapsis is a process by which, during meiosis. there is pairing of two homologous chromosomes.

47. A Chromosome 1

Chromosomes can be classified on the basis of the position of the centromere or their size. The largest and the last completed of all chromosomes is chromosome 1. As human cells are diploid in nature, there are two copies of chromosome 1. It is estimated that chromosome 1 consititues approximately 8% of all DNA in humans. Overall, there are 22 pairs of autosomes and 2 pairs of sex chromosomes (X and Y chromosomes) found in human cells.

48. D S Phase

The cell cycle is a process during which both prokaryotic and eukaryotic cells undergo division and replication. It consists of four phases such as gap 1 (G1), synthesis (S), gap 2 (G2) and mitosis (M). G1, S and G2 phases are together termed 'interphase'. During the G1 phase the cells enlarge in size, and then undergo DNA replication in the S phase. This is followed by the G2 phase characterised by continued cell growth. Finally cell growth stops and the cell enters the M phase which consists of distinct phases such as prophase, metaphase, anaphase, telophase and cytokinesis. G0 is a phase during which the cell is in a resting state.

49. D It means that different genotypes cause the same phenotype but each genotype is associated with very different risks

When different genotypes cause the same phenotype but each genotype is associated with very different phenotypes it is known as genetic heterogeneity. It is either allele based (allelic) or locus based (locus). When different mutations within multiple alleles of the gene at that locus cause the same phenotype, it is called allelic heterogeneity, and when variations in unrelated gene loci cause a single phenotype or disorder it is called locus heterogeneity. Transcription factors control expression of many genes so any mutation in them, known as pleiotropy, can lead to seemingly multiple and unrelated phenotypes, e.g. phenotypic abnormalities in intellectual disability syndromes.

50. B 45, X/46, XX

Most of the women with Turner's syndrome have monosomy X (45,X or 45,XO). There are few who have a chromosomal change in only some of their cells, the mosaic. Therefore, in the presence of mosaicism, there is a mix of cells with the usual two sex chromosomes (either XX or XY) and cells that have only one X chromosome. Turner's syndrome is caused by X-chromosome mosaicism (45,X/46,XX and 45,X/46,XY) and known as mosaic Turner's syndrome which is associated with a high risk of schizophrenia. Around 99% of the fetuses that have Turner's syndrome terminate spontaneously during the first trimester. Trisomy 16 is the most frequent aneuploidy in humans although fetuses do not survive to term. 47,XYY syndrome is associated with an increased risk of autistic disorder spectrum, learning disabilities, and delayed development of speech and language skills.

51. B 25%

The prevalence of schizophrenia in 22q11.2 syndrome is around 23–25%. This syndrome occurs due to deletion of location 22q11.2 on chromosome 22.

Before identification of a deletion in chromosome 22, this syndrome was known by several names such as velocardiofacial syndrome, DiGeorge's syndrome or conotruncal anomaly face syndrome. This syndrome is inherited as an autosomal dominant syndrome. It associated with a 20- to 30-fold increase in the risk of developing schizophrenia and accounts for approximately 1% of all schizophrenia cases.

52. D 46%

The lifetime risk of developing schizophrenia in offspring of both parents who both have schizophrenia is 46%. In the event that one parent has schizophrenia, the offspring has a lifetime risk of 13% (9–16%). If one of the siblings has schizophrenia, the lifetime risk for this illness is estimated to be 10% (8–14%).

53. E Chromosome 6q and 8q

McQueen et al (2005), in a meta-analysis, identified a genome with significant evidence for linkage on the long arm of chromosome 6(6q) for bipolar disorder type 1 and on long arm of chromosome 8(8q) for bipolar disorder types 1 and 2. Other regions on the chromosome that indicate strong evidence for this disorder are 12q and 13q, and chromosome 18. The gene of interest in bipolar disorder is DGKH (diacylglycerol kinase eta) on chromosome 13q14 and a single nucleotide polymorphism on chromosome 16p12.

54. C Panic disorder

Genetic studies indicate that comorbid bipolar disorder and panic disorder may represent a familial subtype of bipolar disorder. Relatives of probands with this familial subtype are more likely to have bipolar type 2 disorder. Panic disorder is present in 15–20% of patients diagnosed with bipolar disorder and is associated with rapid mood swings. In a recent study, offsprings of bipolar affective disorder showed a 5-fold increase in attention deficit hyperactivity disorder and 6-fold increase in anxiety disorder when compared with offsprings of parents not having bipolar affective disorder.

55. A Deletion allele

In depression, the most widely studied candidate gene is *SLC6A4*, which is located on chromosome 17. It encodes for serotonin transporter (ST) which is the target of the selective serotonin reuptake inhibitors. The most common polymorphism in the promoter of the ST gene, which is associated with mood disorders, is the serotonin transporter length polymorphic region (5-HTTLPR). Two alleles commonly found for 5-HTTLPR are the insertion allele (the 'long' allele) and the deletion allele (the 'short' allele). It is the short or deletion allele that has been associated with risk for major depressive disorder and suicidality in patients who are experiencing stressful life events and depressive symptoms. However, environmental factors can counteract the genetic and environmental vulnerability.

56. B Microarray analysis

Comparative genomic hybridisation is a new technology allowing the detection and comparison of submicroscopic regions of chromosomes between patient and a reference sample for DNA. It is also known as chromosomal microarray analysis (CMA). The patient's DNA and the reference DNA are hybridised simultaneously, which will generate a map of DNA copy number changes. CMA detects the unbalanced chromosomal changes, which in turn change the copy number. It does not detect structural chromosome aberrations such as balanced reciprocal translocations or inversions in which there is no change in DNA copy numbers.

57. C Non-additive interaction of alleles at different loci (gene–gene interaction)

Non-additive genetic contribution is due to interaction of alleles within a locus (genetic dominance), interaction of alleles at different loci (gene–gene interaction), also called epistasis, and gene–environment correlation when the individual's genotype is correlated to the environment to which he or she is exposed.

58. D Monozygotic twins reared in the same environment

'Equal environment assumption' assumes that monozygotic (MZ) twins experience a similar environment and are treated more similarly than dizygotic (DZ) twins. One way to reduce this effect is direct observational studies, which have not been used much due to their limitations. Another method is to study twins who are mistaken about their zygosity but it has been shown that true zygosity is a more important influence than perceived zygosity on twin similarity. The best way to examine the influence of environmental sharing in twins is to look at MZ twins who had been reared apart, which is rare but has shown a substantial genetic contribution to psychosis, personality and cognition.

59. A It estimates genetic and environmental contributions using a simple diagrammatic method

Path analysis is basically a simple diagrammatic method used to estimate contribution of genetic and environmental factors. Model fitting serves two purposes: first it tests statistically how a model tries to explain any given data and second compares different models. It comes in various designs and can be applied to complex scenarios including twin data. Multiple regression analysis is also used to analyse twin data. Here the score of a co-twin is predicted from the score of the index twin (the proband). This method also tests if the extent of the genetic contribution of extreme scores for a continuous trait differs from the scores within the normal range.

60. A Approximately 99.5% of cases are a single occurrence in a family

This is inherited as an X-liked dominant condition. It is a pervasive neurodevelopmental disorder with a prevalence of 1:10,000–1:12,000 in girls. There is pervasive growth failure, communication dysfunction and stereotypical movements. Approximately 99.5% of cases are a single occurrence in a family. Gene mutation occurs in the *MECP2* gene. Gaze is the most important way of interacting because other ways of communication are quite compromised. It is the inability to perform motor functions that is the most disabling feature of Rett's syndrome, interfering with every body movement, including eye gaze and speech, although gaze is the most important way of interacting with the environment and patients show their interest by eye pointing. Developmental deviations are apparent by 15 months of age in 50%, by 18 months in 80% and by 2 years in 100%.

61. C Paranoid schizophrenia

This is less familial and has a lower monozygotic twin concordance rate. Also late paraphrenia carries less genetic loading than the early onset type.

62. C 50%

Heritability of social anxiety disorder (SAD) in females is 50%. Monozygotic concordance rate in SAD is 25%, and in dizygotic twins it is 15%. Life events and parental upbringing have an influence. Patients with SAD usually recall their mothers as scared, avoiding social interactions and being overprotective. SAD occurs more often in individuals who undergo stressful social and performance situations early in their lives.

63. E Williams' syndrome

This is the disorder caused by 7q11 microdeletions. It is characterised by infantile hypercalcaemia, supravalvular aortic stenosis, moderate learning disability, hyperacusis and elfin facies. Angelman's syndrome is due to deletion of 15q11 of maternal origin. Prader–Willi syndrome is caused by deletion of a paternally inherited deletion of chromosome 15q11.

64. A Fragile X syndrome

This is caused by expansion of a trinucleotide repeat CGG near the *FMRI* gene. People born with FMRI allele with 200 or more repeats have a learning disability. It is the second most common cause of mental retardation after Down;s syndrome. Fragile X syndrome occurs in 1 in 1000 males and 1 in 2000 females. A repeat of the GAA triplet causes Friedreich's ataxia. The CTG repeat causes myotonic dystrophy. The CAG repeat results in Huntington's disease.

65. C Impulsivity

The P300 amplitude elicited from visual odd ball task is used as an endophenotype of alcohol dependence. This is mainly due to impulsivity. The P300 amplitude is decreased in a son who is born to a father with alcohol problems, but has no problem with alcohol. Disorders such as attention deficit hyperactivity disorder, oppositional defiant disorder, antisocial personality disorder and conduct disorder, in which impulsivity is a feature, also show a reduced P300 amplitude. This suggests that P300, although a phenotype that is highly heritable, is linked to intermediate phenotype (impulsivity) rather than alcohol dependence.

66. B Gottesman and Shields

They proposed the concept of 'endophenotypes'. Falconer is associated with work in quantitative genetics. Gregor Mendel is well known for his work on laws of mendelian inheritance. John and Lewis were the pioneers in developing the concept of endophenotype. Michael Rutter is well known in the field of child psychiatry and genetics in autism; he was called the 'father of child psychology'.

67. A Endophenotypes and the illness co-segregate

For a biomarker to be called an endophenotype, it has to satisfy a few criteria such as heritability, association with illness in the population, manifestation irrespective of state of illness (illness present or absent), higher presence in non-affected family members compared with the general population, in addition to co-segregation with illness in families.

68. E *GABRA2* gene

Collaborative studies on the genetics of alcoholism reported an association with chromosomes 4 and 15. Further analysis provided evidence for the gene for the GABA-receptor α-subunit gene (GABRA2 gene) in chromosome 4 to be associated with alcoholism.

69. B Common variants in the genes neuregulin-1 and dysbindin, and the D-amino acid oxidase activator contribute a small increase in risk for schizophrenia

There is considerable debate about the exact genetic architecture of schizophrenia. Common variants in the genes neuregulin-1 and dysbindin, and the D-amino acid oxidase activator confer a small increase in the risk for schizophrenia. Recent whole-genome association analyses suggests that multiple low-penetrance common variants contribute to risk for schizophrenia. Common high-penetrance variants have not generally been found in the recent studies. Monozygotic co-twins are only 50% concordant for the disorder. Dizygotic co-twins are 10% concordant for schizophrenia. There is evidence of considerable variation between populations in susceptibility genes and variants.

70. C There is no role for environmental factors in the development of disorder

In twin studies, two types of environmental influences are observed. They are called shared environment and non-shared environment. Shared-environmental factors include all non-genetic factors that make the family members similar. Non-shared environmental factors are environmental influences that differentiate one family member from the others, including the measurement effect. In twin studies, if both monozygotic and dizygotic correlations are substantial and do not differ by zygosity, then shared environmental influences are indicated.

71. D Huntington's disease

Linkage analysis is useful in identifying genes in conditions such as cystic fibrosis and Huntington's disease. These illnesses are due to one gene disorder in which a rough position of the gene in respect of known genetic markers is easier to identify compared with a complex illness involving several genes and/or non-gene-related factors. This procedure of rough location of disease gene is called linkage analysis.

72. B Living in urban areas

Heritability is defined as the proportion of total phenotype variance accounted for by gene effects. Heritability is influenced by environmental factors that are either less controlled or less structured. Some of these environmental factors are being single, no religious background, living in urban areas and environment with less opportunity to express behaviour differences. This helps us to understand the influence of genes and environment in different circumstances and variations in the estimates of heritability in different settings for the same disorder.

73. B Structured situations are those that provide relatively unambiguous cues to guide behaviour

Situations with fewer structures become ambiguous. In structured situations causes of behaviour are more situational and, where the situation is more ambiguous, the behaviour is more likely to result from individual dispositions. In less structured situations, because there are few salient cues in the environment, individuals must rely to a greater extent on their own disposition to guide behaviour.

74. D 6%

The total prevalence of mental health disorder in patients with a learning disability is generally higher than in the general population. Several population-based studies have highlighted this increased prevalence.

Specific phobia: 6%
Generalised anxiety disorder: 6%
Agoraphobia: 1.5%
Obsessive–compulsive disorder: 2.5%

75. B High education level

Several personal and social factors influence the risk of suicide in schizophrenia. Some of these factors that increase risk are:

Higher levels of education
High IQ
Good insight into illness
Poor compliance
Aggression and impulsivity
Living alone or not living with family
Recent loss
Family history of suicide.

76. B Depression

Intermittent depressive symptoms are common in schizophrenia. The presence of a depressive disorder increases the risk of suicide in schizophrenia. Depression can be missed due to negative symptoms of illness or side effects of neuroleptics. Loss of emotional contact, loss of energy and inertia are common in both. Hopelessness and a pessimistic view of the future are important signs that suggest depression. It is not felt that delusions or hallucinations markedly increase the suicide risk.

77. E White ethnicity

The risk for suicide is considered highest in the following:

White ethnicity
Early course of illness, especially within first year of diagnosis
First episode in older age group patients (two recent studies)
Soon after diagnosis
Those who attempt suicide
Number of psychiatric admissions
Within 1 week of discharge from hospital
High educational level/high IQ/high level of functioning before illness
Good insight into illness

78. A China

This is the only country that has higher female than male suicide rates. The ratio of male:female suicide was 0.78 in 1991 and 0.91 in 2001. This creates an ecological fallacy, which means that what is true at the aggregate level (population level) should be true for the individual level.

79. B Life-time prevalence is 4/1000

Saha et al (2005) carried out systematic review of prevalence of schizophrenia. The authors of the study concluded that there is no statistical difference between male and female, or urban, rural and mixed site prevalence rates. Developing countries had a lower prevalence rate. However, migrants and homeless people had a higher rate of schizophrenia. Definitions of migrants in the studies are variable.

Life-time prevalence – 4/1000
Point prevalence – 3.3/1000
Median prevalence – 4.6/1000
Life-time morbid risk – 7.2/1000

80. E Insidious onset

Morgan et al (2006) in a study of aetiology and ethnicity of schizophrenia and other psychoses studied the clinical and social determinants of duration of untreated psychosis (DUP) in patients with first episode psychosis. The study found that insidious/gradual onset of psychosis was a significant predictor of DUP and associated with a longer DUP. Similarly, unemployment was associated with a longer DUP, although this association was not as strong. Short DUP was associated with acute onset and family involvement in seeking independent help. Affective psychosis may be related to shorter DUP, although this was not statistically significant. Similarly, Compton et al (2008) concluded that patients with insidious/gradual onset were 50% less likely to be hospitalised.

81. E 5%

According to a national survey in England and Wales by Meehan et al (2006), of all the people convicted of homicide, 5% had schizophrenia. Of these, about 50% had been ill for <12 months and in the month before the offence. About 50% had shown some change in the delusional belief (emotional response, intensity or conviction). About a third (28%) had no previous contact with psychiatric services.

82. B 50%

Psychotic symptoms occur in around 50% of patients with delirium. Delusions are poorly formed and less stereotyped; they are usually fleeting, fragmentary and persecutory, e.g. being harassed by medical staff on the ward, but they may sometimes be grandiose. Depersonalisation and delusional perception may occur. Hallucinations and illusions are usually visual although they may be tactile or auditory.

83. A Abnormal motor and speech development before 2 years

The incidence of schizophrenia increases linearly with the decrement of IQ. There are problems with development of motor and speech before 2 years of age and soft neurological signs such as poor motor control, balance and coordination are present along with non-right-handedness. Severe hypoxic perinatal brain damage, low birthweight (<2500 g) and high birthweight (>4000 g) may also occur. Urbanisation contributes by causation (the breeder effect) and by attracting vulnerable people (the drift effect). Also the risk is high if the city is large and individuals living longer in cities have a high risk. Social class also affects via social causation (breeder effect) and social selection, i.e. drift.

84. E Withdrawal of antipsychotics

The best short-term predictor of relapse is withdrawal of medication, usually due to non-compliance. Other choices are also short-term predictors. Medium- to long-term predictors with poor prognosis are male, single, premorbid social withdrawal and insidious onset.

85. A East of England

As per the government office regions in England 2000–2009, the male suicide rate in England was highest in the northern regions and lowest in the east of England and London. There was no clear pattern in regional suicide rates in females.

86. C 50%

More than half of patients with mental illness smoke tobacco. It has been noticed that patients with emotional disorders and conduct disorder have four and six times increased rates of smoking, respectively, compared with the general population. Nearly 70% of inpatients on a mental health ward, 80% of prisoners with mental health problems and nearly 60–80% of those on methadone who attend clinics smoke tobacco. Hence, smoking is noted to be significantly high in people with mental illness compared with the general population.

87. D 1 every 40 seconds

This an estimated figure by the World Health Organization.

88. B General health questionnaire

This is a self-rating scale that was developed by Professor David Goldberg. It is a screening tool to detect psychiatric disorders in community disorders and non-psychiatric settings such as primary care or general practice. The other options in the question are interview-rated scales.

89. C Incidence

This is a measure of disease frequency. It is defined as follows:

Incidence — cumulative incidence/incidence risk/incidence proportion

— incidence density/incidence rate/person–time incidence

— incidence odds

Prevalence — point prevalence

— period prevalence

— prevalence odds

Measure of association

Risk difference/attributable risk/absolute risk reduction

Number needed to treat

Odds ratio.

90. E Montgomery–Asberg depression rating scale

The Montgomery–Asberg depression rating scale is a clinician-rated scale having a 10-item checklist. It is most sensitive to change in depression symptoms and widely used in drug trials.

Beck's depression inventory: mainly self-administered. Mainly used to measure attitude and symptoms that are characteristic of depression.

Bech–Rafaelsen melancholia scale: a clinician-rated scale. Used to measure the severity of symptoms and also changes in depressive state during treatment.

Major depression inventory: is a self-rated questionnaire by patient for identification of depression.

Hamilton depression rating scale or HAM-D: clinician-rated scale to measure severity of depressive illness.

91. C Galbraith's plot

This is used to identify studies that contribute most to heterogeneity in meta-analytical statistics.

Fixed effect analysis is a method in which two or more studies are combined in a meta-analytic study. In this case there is low heterogeneity.

The other three statistical measures: log rank test, Cox's proportional hazard analysis and Kaplan–Meier method, are used to perform survival analysis in a study.

92. A Bech–Rafaelsen scale

In studies that intend to investigate, both depression and mania, Bech–Rafaelsen scale for both mania and melancholia may be the most appropriate. Of course, a combination of depression and mania rating scales can be used in a research study. Hopelessness scale is used in studies for suicide.

93. A Defensive functioning scale

This is a rating scale used to assess personality by evaluating a person's coping strategies and categorising his or her defence mechanisms into seven levels. Global assessment of relational functioning is used to evaluate the family environment and other relationships. Million clinical mini-inventory (MCMI) is a personality assessment scale developed by Theodore Millon, intended to provide insight into a person's psychopathology; it has 175 questions (Yes/No questions). The Minnesota multiphasic personality inventory is a semi-structured personality assessment interview relevant to the DSM-IV. Rorschach's test by Hermann Rorschach is a projective test for assessment of personality and emotional functioning. The thematic apperception test is another projective test for personality assessment designed by Murray and Morgan.

94. B Intact procedural memory

The defining features of the amnestic syndrome include intact immediate memory, intact intelligence, intact semantic memory, severe and permanent anterograde memory, and intact procedural memory

95. B Impairment in executive functioning

Neuropsychological abnormalities are widely reported in people with schizophrenia; they include impairments in learning, memory and executive functioning.

96. E Viscerotonic

In the early twentith century, Sheldon described a link between personality and build, summarised in **Table 2.7**. However, later on more systematic and controlled research studies failed to support his theory of linking body type and personality.

Table 2.7 Body shape and temperament		
Sheldon's somatotype and temperament	Cluster of traits	Body shape
Endomorphic body type: viscerotonic temperament	Love of food, comfort, people and affection	Plump
Mesomorphic body type: somatotonic temperament	High desire for physical adventure, risk taking and muscular activities	Muscular
Ectomorphic body type: cerebrotonic temperament	Emotional restraint, self-consciousness, preference for solitude and privacy	Lean

97. D Maladaptive

The general diagnostic criteria of personality disorder include: they appear in late childhood or adolescence, and they are not secondary to other mental disorder and brain disease. They are pervasive and cause distress to self and others. There is personal distress or an adverse impact on the personal environment.

98. D Irresponsible attitude

An irresponsible attitude that is persistent is one of the criteria in the ICD-10 for the diagnosis of dissocial personality disorder. In addition, patients who have dissocial personality disorder take no notice of social standards, rules or duties, thereby disregarding them. They are insensitive to other people's feelings and are unable to empathise. They are not able to maintain long-term relationships. They can get easily frustrated and be involved in violent and aggressive outbursts.

They blame others rather than self which can lead to conflict with others. They do not have increased interest in sexual activity in particular. Persistent irritability and conduct disorder in adolescence are not essential for diagnosis according to the ICD-10. However, their presence does complete the clinical picture of dissocial personality disorder.

99. D Histrionic personality disorder

Psychoanalytical theory processes propose that histrionic personality disorder originates in the oedipal phase of development (3–5 years of age). This is when an overly eroticised relationship with the opposite sex parent is unduly encouraged and the child feels that the consequence of this excitement is the loss of the relationship of the same-sex parent.

100. B DBT appears to result in reduced suicide attempts

According to Linehan et al (2007), patients with borderline personality receiving DBT were half as likely to attempt suicide, required less hospitalisation for suicidal intention and had lower medical risk after suicide attempts or self-harm. More patients remained in treatment and required less inpatient admission and emergency care. Studies of DBT suggest that its effectiveness cannot be attributed completely to general factors associated with expert psychotherapy.

101. B Almost three-quarters of children are found to be securely attached

The strange situation experiment was devised by Ainsworth and Wittig in 1969. Three types were observed during the experiment.

Table 2.8 Types of attachments

Category	Description	%
Type A: anxious avoidant	Baby largely ignores mother because of indifference towards her. No or few signs of distress when mother leaves. Ignores her when she arrives. Comforted as easily by stranger as by mother	15
Type B: securely attached	Baby plays happily when mother is present. Distressed when mother leaves and play is reduced. Stranger can provide only limited comfort	70
Type C: anxious resistant	Baby cries more, very distressed when mother leaves. Seeks comfort when mother returns but also shows anger and resists contact. Resists strangers' contact, i.e. treats mother and stranger differently	15

Main identified type D: insecure–disorganised in which the baby lacks goals, shows contradictory behaviour and even shows fear of the mother. Type D has been linked to infant maltreatment, hostile caregiving, maternal loss through separation/divorce/death and maternal depression.

102. D Object permanence develops in the preoperational stage

Piaget divided cognitive development in a child into four stages.

Table 2.9 Piaget's stages of cognitive development

Stage	Age	Abilities/development
Sensorimotor	0–2 years	Object permanence by 18 months
Preoperational	2–7 years	Subdivisions: preconceptual (2–4 years), intuitive (4–7 years) Synthetic thought, transductive reasoning, animism, centration, egocentrism, conservation
Concrete operational	7–11 years	Performs logical operations, relativism, onset of seriation, decline in egocentrism
Formal operational	11 years onwards	Manipulating ideas or propositions. Can think hypothetically, hypothetico-deductive reasoning

103. E Powerful demands in the form of heterosexual desires in the genital stage

According to Freud a child's sexuality develops through the following stages.

Table 2.10 Stages of psychosexual development

Stage	Age	Development
Oral	0–1 years	Pleasure derived from sucking for its own sake. Major activities include sucking, swallowing and mouthing
Anal	1–3 years	Child undergoes potty training, parents love is no more unconditional and they are seen as authority figures
Phallic	3–5/6 years	Pleasure is derived from masturbation. Beginning of Oedipus complex. Super-ego and sex role are acquired
Latency	5/6 to puberty	Sexual energies are repressed and channelised. Id, ego and super-ego balance is greatest the first time in child's development
Genital	Puberty– maturity	Harmony in a child's personality is disrupted by the id's powerful new demands in the form of heterosexual desires

104. D Preconventional morality corresponds to the preoperational stage in Piaget's development

It was Piaget who differentiated two types of moral orientation. Heteronomous morality is seen at age 5–9 years and signifies working on another's laws or rules. Autonomous moral orientation starts after 10 years of age and is subject to its own laws or rules.

Table 2.11 Kohlberg's theory of moral development

Kohlberg's levels and stages	Age group	Corresponding Piaget's stages
Level 1: preconventional morality		
Stage 1: punishment and obedience orientation	Mostly < 9 years	Preoperational stage 2–7 years
Stage 2: instrumental relativist orientation		
Level 2: conventional morality		
Stage 3: interpersonal concordance orientation	Adolescent	Concrete operational stage
Stage 4: maintaining social order orientation	years–adulthood	7–11 years
Level 3: post conventional morality		
Stage 5: social contract–legalistic orientation	10–15 % adults,	Formal operational stage 11
Stage 6: universal ethical principles orientation	> 30 years age	years and above

105. B Gender consistency

According to Kohlberg, children acquire understanding of their own sexual identity in three stages.

Table 2.12 Kohlberg's stages of sexual identity

Stage	Age range	Development
Stage 1: gender labelling or basic gender identity	18 months to 3 years	Child learns to identify own gender, but can struggle to realise that boys become men as adults. The knowledge is fragile
Stage 2: gender stability	3–5 years	Most children recognise that gender remains stable for rest of their lives. But their understanding of gender remains at superficial/physical level
Stage 3: gender constancy or consistency	6–7 years	Children realise that gender is permanent and remains so over time and situations. Their understanding is now beyond physical characteristics, e.g. women can have short hair

106. E It was originally called 'the conversational model'

Psychodynamic interpersonal therapy (PIP), which is also known as the conversational model was developed by Hobson. It has seven components. These are:

1. Explanatory rationale
2. Shared understanding
3. Staying with feelings
4. Focusing on difficult feelings
5. Gaining insight
6. Sequencing of interventions
7. Making changes.

PIP can be a short- or long-term intervention. It has evidence for the management of depression and somatisation.

107. A Faulty procedures include snags, traps and dilemmas

Cognitive–analytic therapy (CAT) is a brief therapy that integrates cognitive–behavioural therapy, psychodynamic psychotherapy and recent developments in the field of cognitive psychology. It was developed by Ryle.

There are two models in the theoretical structure:

1. Procedural sequence model: to understand aim-directed actions. Any aim-directed activity follows the steps listed here:
   - Aim generation
   - Environmental evaluation
   - Plan formulation
   - Action
   - Evaluation
   - Procedural revision.

   The faulty procedural sequences that occur in any aim-directed activity keep recurring. Faulty procedures include traps, snags and dilemmas.

2. Restricted role repertoire: there is a restriction in the range of procedural sequences available that is seen more often with childhood adversity such as abuse.

108. A One of the techniques is to emphasise personal choice and control

Motivational interviewing is a patient directive approach that helps to achieve behaviour change. There are many applications in psychiatry, particularly where there is resistance to change.

There are four main principles:

1. Empathy
2. Create a discrepancy in the attitude/behaviour
3. Remove resistance without confrontation
4. Support self-efficiency to achieve change.

109. E Systematic desensitisation represents a form of counter-conditioning

Behaviour therapy is based on classic conditioning whereas behaviour modification is based on operant conditioning. Systematic desensitisation represents a form of counter-conditioning and the key principle involved here is reciprocal inhibition. In a review of studies, flooding has been found to be the most universally effective of all techniques to treat phobias.

110. E The last two stages are unlikely to be available in most public healthcare settings

DBT has four stages of treatment for borderline personality disorder. Stages 1 and 2 are usually available in public healthcare settings. Stage 1 is most readily available in a public healthcare setting and the focus is to help an individual to control his or her own behaviour, which may interfere with therapy, and reduce self-harming and suicidal behaviours. Stage 2 focuses on processing of emotions related to past trauma and experiences. Stage 3 focuses on addressing the issue of solving problems of everyday life, such as job, relationship, social interaction and learning techniques to deal with them. Stage 4 focuses on the ability to experience joy that is lasting. However, stages 3 and 4 of DBT are unlikely to be available in most public healthcare settings.

111. D Multisystemic therapy

The presentation is probably due to antisocial behaviour in a young offender. In this case, a multisystemic therapy is recommended. This is an intensive family- and community-based intervention and follows a strict model over 4–6 months. It has a good evidence base for its use in juvenile offenders who have fewer out-of-home placements, reduced offending and less substance-related offending.

112. C Shaping

Behavioural techniques derived from earlier work through classic and operant conditioning are assessed through:

1. Interviews
2. Rating scales
3. Diary

The interventions used increase or decrease behaviour.

Table 2.13 Shaping

Interventions to	
Increase behaviour	**Decrease behaviour**
• Positive reinforcement	• Stimulus control
• Social rewards	• Punishment
• Tangible rewards	• Time out
• Application of rewards	• Response cost
• Schedules of reinforcement	• Overcorrection
• Negative reinforcements	• Differential reinforcement of other behaviour or incompatible behaviour
• Token systems	• Graded exposure/systematic desensitisation
• Shaping	• Flooding
• Premack's principle	• Modelling
• Modelling	• Role playing
• Prompting	

113. C Eye movement desensitisation and reprocessing

The man presents with post-traumatic stress disorder. The psychological therapy of choice is eye movement desensitisation and reprocessing that is a variant of behavioural therapy. The patient is asked to recall the event that is traumatic while a relaxed state is being induced by the therapist. This is done by the patient focusing on the therapist's voice and movement of fingers.

Trauma-focused cognitive therapy and exposure therapy can also be used.

114. C Moral conflicts happen between the super-ego and the ego

According to Freud's psychoanalytic theory, personality comprises three parts: the id, ego and super-ego. The id is governed by pleasure principle and is the infantile, presocialised part of personality. Two major id instincts are sexuality and aggression. Ego is considered the 'executive' of the personality and is associated with the reality principle. It deals with planning, decision-making, rational and logical thinking, and in deferred gratification. The super-ego is considered the moral 'policeman' that threatens the ego with punishment.

115. E Systems training for emotional predictability and problem solving is a CBT-based skills development package

Systems training for emotional predictability and problem solving is delivered as 2-hourly sessions over a duration of 20 weeks. It is based on a CBT model and focuses on development of skills in patients with borderline personality disorder. CBT for borderline personality disorder differs from other CBT models in that it focuses on 'schemas' and deals with previous experiences rather than the 'here and now'. The number of CBT sessions required for this disorder is relatively more than axis I disorders and may range from 9 weeks to 36 weeks. Complementary therapy and art therapy have a limited evidence base and are not mainstream therapies used in the NHS.

116. B It is delivered over 20 weeks

There is limited randomised controlled trial (RCT) evidence for individual psychological interventions. There is weak RCT evidence for CAT (in young people), and systems training for emotional predictability and problem solving (STEPPS) in improving general functioning and reducing self-harm. Non-RCT evidence shows positive outcomes and that it is well accepted by patients. CBT, schema-focused psychotherapy and individual psychotherapy have not shown much benefits.

STEPPS is a CBT-based skills development package presented in 2-hour sessions for patients with borderline personality disorder. The therapy is delivered over 20 weeks with a 2-hour session for family members and significant others. It is designed to be used to complement other treatments.

117. E Snags

Anthony Ryle developed CAT.

There are two models in the theoretical structure:

- Procedural sequence model: the faulty procedural sequences that occur in any aim-directed activity keep recurring. Faulty procedures include traps, snags and dilemmas.
- Restricted role repertoire: there is a restriction in the range of procedural sequences available which is seen more often with childhood adversity such as abuse.

118. A Aims of psychological therapy include reduction in mood fluctuations and maintaining a stable mental state

Psychological therapy in bipolar affective disorder (BPAD) focuses on reducing the chance of relapse of illness and improving levels of functioning. It further aims to reduce the symptoms and fluctuations in mood. There has been only one study of medication adherence and one study on psychological therapy for people with comorbid substance use disorder. Formal therapies such as CBT or psychodynamic psychotherapy are rarely offered to children with BPAD.

119. A Family interventions should focus on how the disorder impacts on family relationships

There is a small but consistent evidence base for efficacy of family interventions. Such interventions should focus on how the disorder impacts on family relationships. Parents should be encouraged to take a central role in the early stages of treatment, supporting the child's efforts to eat. Seeing parents and young people together and separately may show benefits. Issues such as confidentiality and consent must be considered carefully and not be simply overridden by clinicians or parents.

120. B Delusional beliefs

One of the studies published in 1997, the London–East Anglia randomised controlled trial on CBT in psychosis, suggested that there was cognitive flexibility in patients who had delusional beliefs. CBT was effective in producing positive outcomes in psychosis with patients experiencing delusional beliefs.

121. A Arbitrary inference

Projection bias is a tendency to unconsciously assume that others (or one's future selves) share one's current emotional states, thoughts and values. According to Beck's theory of depression there were four main cognitive biases. Arbitrary inference refers to drawing conclusions in the absence of sufficient or any evidence. Selective abstraction refers to conclusions drawn on the basis of just one of the many elements in a situation. Overgeneralisation refers to deriving sweeping conclusions on the basis of a single and usually trivial event. Magnification and minimisations are exaggerations in evaluating performance.

122. A Cognitive-behavioural therapy

Although there are no specific definitions for high- or low-intensity psychological treatments, interventions that use less resources are considered low-intensity treatments. For example, in the case of non-facilitated self-help virtually no resources are used. Usually low-intensity psychological therapies are often delivered and/or supported by mental health workers. Although CBT can also be 'low intensity', compared with the other options, it is the best possible answer.

123. B SRRS assumes that any change in life is by definition stressful

The social readjustment rating scale (SRRS) was developed by Holmes and Rahe (1967), which examined 5000 patients and made a list of 43 life events. The life change unit (LCU) score of > 150 in 1 year is classed as a life crisis, 150–199 as mild, 200–299 as moderate and > 300 as a major crisis. Some of the mean values in SRRS are: death of a spouse 100 (highest value), jail term 63, marriage 50, son/daughter leaving home 29, minor violations of the law 11 (lowest value).

Chapter 3

Test questions: 3

Questions: MCQs

For each question, select one answer option.

NEUROSCIENCES: NEUROANATOMY

1. A 58-year-old man presented to the accident and emergency department with clinical features suggestive of an occlusion of the right medial striate branch of the anterior cerebral artery. Which of the following is correct?

    A   Akinetic mutism
    B   Apathy with memory loss
    C   Ideomotor apraxia
    D   Paresis of face and arm
    E   Tactile anomia

2. What is the most likely neurological damage caused by the lacunar infarct of the genu of the internal capsule?

    A   Dysarthria–clumsy hand syndrome
    B   Broca's aphasia
    C   Pure motor hemiparesis
    D   Pure sensory syndrome
    E   Wernicke's aphasia

3. Which of the following functions is most likely to be affected by a lesion in the non-dominant hemisphere?

    A   Body-image formation
    B   Left–right disorientation
    C   Understanding of non-verbal communication
    D   Verbal memory
    E   Writing ability

4. Which part of the brain is related to alterations in memory?

    A   Frontal lobe
    B   Frontoparietal lobe
    C   Occipital lobe
    D   Parietal lobe
    E   Temporal lobe

5. Which of the following lobe lesions is associated with difficulties in calculation, and perceptual and spatial orientation?

    A   Dominant frontal lobe
    B   Dominant occipital lobe

    C   Dominant parietal lone
    D   Non-dominant parietal lobe
    E   Non-dominant temporal lobe

6. Which of the following is a part of the limbic lobe nuclei?

    A   Amygdaloid nucleus
    B   Corpus striatum
    C   Cingulate gyrus
    D   Dendate nuclues
    E   Septal nucleus

7. Which of the following is a part of the basal ganglia?

    A   Amygdaloid nucleus
    B   Corpus striatum
    C   Cingulate gyrus
    D   Dendate gyrus
    E   Visual association cortex

8. Which of the following cranial nerves innervate intrinsic muscles of larynx?

    A   Accessory nerve
    B   Hypoglossal nerve
    C   Trochlear nerve
    D   Vagus nerve
    E   Vestibulocochlear nerve

9. Where is the entire nervous system derived from?

    A   Neural crest
    B   Neural folds
    C   Neural plate
    D   Neural pores
    E   Neural tube

10. When is the formation of the neural tube completed during gestation?

    A   First week
    B   Second week
    C   Third week
    D   Fourth week
    E   Fifth week

11. Which of the following structures include the tectum?

    A   Diencephalon
    B   Mesencephalon
    C   Prosencephalon
    D   Rhombencephalon
    E   Telencephalon

12. Which of the following structures differentiate into striatum and pallidum?

    A   Diencephalon
    B   Mesencephalon
    C   Metencephalon
    D   Rhombencephalon
    E   Telencephalon

13. Which of the following structures is responsible for origin of cerebellum?

    A   Diencephalon
    B   Mesencephalon
    C   Prosencephalon
    D   Rhombencephalon
    E   Telencephalon

NEUROSCIENCES: NEUROPATHOLOGY

14. A 45-year-old man was diagnosed with frontotemporal dementia. Which of the following histopathological changes is most likely to be seen in his brain?

    A   Global brain atrophy
    B   Knife blade gyri, ventricular enlargement
    C   Reactive astrocytosis
    D   Sulcal widening
    E   Ventricular enlargement

15. A 62-year-old man was diagnosed with vascular dementia. Which of the following represents the histopathological changes of his condition?

    A   Arteriosclerotic changes in major arteries
    B   Changes including infarction and ischaemia
    C   Local or generalised brain atrophy
    D   Sulcal widening
    E   Ventricular enlargement

16. Which of the following conditions is classified as both a tauopathy and an amyloidopathy?

    A   Alzheimer's disease
    B   Down's syndrome
    C   Frontotemporal dementia
    D   Pick's disease
    E   Progressive supranuclear palsy

17. A 72-year-old man was diagnosed with Alzheimer's disease according to the criteria of the consortium to establish a registry for Alzheimer's disease (CERAD). Which of the following is not considered a part of the CERAD criteria?

    A   Assessment of amyloid plaque density
    B   Brain weight
    C   Pallor of substantia nigra
    D   Prion deposition
    E   Ventricular dilatation

18. A 32-year-old man presented with glial nodules, rhabdomyoma of the heart and subungal angiofibroma. What is the most likely diagnosis?

    A   Ataxia telangiectasia
    B   Klinefelter's syndrome
    C   Sturge–Weber syndrome
    D   Tuberous sclerosis
    E   Von Hippel–Lindau disease

19. Which of the following is the most common cerebral tumour?

    A   Gliomas
    B   Haemangioblastomas
    C   Medulloblastomas
    D   Meningeal tumours
    E   Pituitary adenomas

NEUROSCIENCES: NEUROPHYSIOLOGY

20. What is the average number of sleep cycles that a person goes through during the night?

    A   0–2
    B   3–5
    C   6–9
    D   10–12
    E   12–15

21. According to the Erlanger and Gasser classification, which of the following nerve fibres have the maximum conduction velocity?

    A   Aα
    B   Aβ
    C   Aδ
    D   Aγ
    E   B

22. Which of the following receptors is linked with moderate type of transmitter system?

    A α-amino-3-hydroxy-5-methyl-4-isoxazolepropionic acid
    B γ-Aminobutyric acid A (GABA-A)
    C   GABA-B
    D   Kainate
    E   N-Methyl-D-aspartate

23. Which of the following is a metabotrophic receptor?

    A   GABA-A
    B   Glutamate (AMPA/K)
    C   Glycine
    D   Histamine (H$_1$, H$_2$, H$_3$)
    E   Purines

24. In the membrane transport system, there is a protein that withdraws the vesicle membrane from the synaptic cleft. What is the name of this protein?

    A   Actin
    B   Calmodulin
    C   Clathrin
    D   Dynamin
    E   Synaptophysin

25. Which of the following is the action of calmodulin in the transmitter transport system?

    A   Brings vesicle into contact with the presynaptic membrane
    B   Creates the membrane fusion pore

C   Expels vesicle content into the synaptic cleft
D   Pinches the neck of the developing vesicles to completes its separation
E   Withdraws the vesicle membrane from the synaptic cleft

26. Which type of nerve fibre innervates deep pressure sensors in muscles?

A   Ia
B   Ib
C   II
D   III
E   IV

27. Which type of nerve fibre has a velocity of 25–70 m/s?

A   Ia
B   Ib
C   II
D   III
E   IV

NEUROSCIENCES: NEUROENDOCRINOLOGY

28. Which hormone is secreted by the posterior pituitary?

A   Antidiuretic hormone
B   Adrenocorticotrophic hormone
C   Growth hormone
D   Luteinising hormone
E   Prolactin

NEUROSCIENCES: NEUROCHEMISTRY

29. Which of the following enzymes converts dopamine to noradrenaline?

A   Acetyl-coenzyme A
B   Alcohol dehydrogenase
C   Aldehyde dehydrogenase
D   Choline acetyl transferase
E   Dopamine β-hydroxylase

30. Which of the following enzymes is responsible for the degradation of monoamines in presynaptic neuron vesicles?

A   Acetyl-coenzyme A
B   Alcohol dehydrogenase
C   Aldehyde dehydrogenase
D   Choline acetyl transferase
E   Catechol-O-methyltransferase

31. Which of the following is a precursor in the synthesis of noradrenaline?

A   Choline
B   L-Tryptophan
C   L-Tyrosine

D   Dopamine β-hydroxylase
E   Histidine

32. Which of the following best describes dopamine?

    A   Degraded by dopa decarboxylase
    B   Immediate precursor of L-dopa
    C   Receptors are ionotropic
    D   Stored in postsynaptic complex
    E   Synthesised from L-tyrosine

33. Which of the following enzymes is responsible for the degradation of monoamines in the synapse?

    A   Acetyl-coenzyme A
    B   Alcohol dehydrogenase
    C   Aldehyde dehydrogenase
    D   Choline acetyl transferase
    E   Catechol-O-methyltransferase

34. Which enzyme is inhibited by disulfiram?

    A   Acetyl-coenzyme A
    B   Alcohol dehydrogenase
    C   Aldehyde dehydrogenase
    D   Choline acetyl transferase
    E   Dopamine β-hydroxylase

NEUROSCIENCES: NEUROIMAGING

35. Leigh's disease is often characterised by symmetrical necrosis manifested on CT or MRI. What part of the brain is involved in this process?

    A   Basal ganglia
    B   Cerebellum
    C   Frontal lobe
    D   Parietal lobe
    E   Temporal lobe

36. Which of the following imaging technique involves use of radioactive compounds to study regional differences in blood flow in the brain?

    A   CT
    B   fMRI
    C   MRI
    D   Positron emission tomography
    E   Single photon emission computed tomography

37. A 55-year-old man was diagnosed with dementia with Lewy bodies. Which of the following findings is likely to be observed on SPECT?

    A   Reduced blood flow in frontal lobe
    B   Reduced blood flow in parietal lobe
    C   Reduced blood flow in temporal lobes
    D   Reduced blood flow in occipital lobe
    E   Variable and multifocal areas of reduced blood flow

38. Which of the following changes is seen on neuroimaging in patients with schizophrenia?

A   Enlarged medial temporal lobes
B   Increased activity in the frontal lobe
C   Reduced phospholipids in the frontal lobe
D   Reduced ventricular size
E   Striatal hypodominergic activity

39. A medical student wanted to know what was used in MRI to construct images of tissues. What would you tell him?

A   Blood oxygenation level-dependent technique
B   Gamma rays
C   Protons
D   Radioisotopes
E   X-ray imaging

PSYCHOPHARMACOLOGY: PHARMACOKINETICS

40. Which of the following is a risk factor for antidepressant-induced hyponatremia?

A   Diabetes mellitus
B   Hyperthyroidism
C   Male
D   Obesity
E   Young age

41. A 20-year-old male student of Asian ethnicity drank alcohol for the first time in his life. As soon as he had a glass of beer he developed tachycardia, facial flushing, sweating, and muscle weakness. What is the most likely reason?

A   Aldehyde dehydrogenase 1 deficiency
B   Aldehyde dehydrogenase 2 deficiency
C   Aldehyde dehydrogenase 3 deficiency
D   Aldehyde dehydrogenase 4 deficiency
E   Aldehyde dehydrogenase 5 deficiency

42. A 44-year-old man diagnosed with bipolar affective disorder has recently started taking lithium carbonate 200 mg twice a day. Which of the following blood tests will give a good indication of serum lithium levels?

A   A blood test done 12 hours after the last night dose on day 2 of starting lithium carbonate
B   A blood test done 12 hours after the last night dose on day 10 of starting lithium carbonate and delaying the morning dose till the blood test is done
C   A blood test done 13 hours after the last night dose on day 10 of starting lithium carbonate while administering the morning dose on time
D   A blood test done 15 hours after the last night dose on day 10 of starting lithium carbonate while administering the morning dose on time
E   A blood test done 9 hours after the last night dose on day 10 of starting lithium carbonate while administering the morning dose on time

43. A 25-year-old man has achieved complete remission of depressive illness on treatment with paroxetine. He stopped taking paroxetine abruptly without seeking medical advice and experienced tremors, sweating and electric shock-like sensations in his legs. What is the most likely diagnosis?

A   Alcohol withdrawal
B   Discontinuation syndrome

    C   Panic disorder
    D   Relapse of depressive episode
    E   Stroke

PSYCHOPHARMACOLOGY: PHARMACODYNAMICS

44. A 45-year-old woman has recurrent depressive disorder on fluoxetine 60 mg with limited benefit. You had a discussion with the patient to stop fluoxetine and start mirtazapine. According to NICE guidelines, which of the following is the most appropriate way to do it?

    A   Cross-taper fluoxetine with mirtazapine cautiously
    B   Reduce fluoxetine to 40 mg and start mirtazapine 15 mg
    C   Reduce fluoxetine to 20 mg and start mirtazapine 15 mg
    D   Stop fluoxetine and start mirtazapine
    E   Stop fluoxetine, wait for 4–7 days and start mirtazapine

45. Which of the following statements about treatment during breastfeeding is correct?

    A   Diazepam is preferred over lorazepam for anxiety
    B   Fluoxetine is the preferred antidepressant drug
    C   Lamotrigine is preferred for bipolar depression
    D   Lithium is preferred as a mood stabiliser
    E   Olanzapine is the preferred antipsychotic drug

46. A 68-year-old man diagnosed with Alzheimer's disease was started on memantine. He reported sudden worsening of cognitive symptoms 3 weeks after starting the treatment. What is the most likely reason for this?

    A   Nicotine acetylcholine receptor antagonism
    B N-methyl-D-aspartate (NMDA) receptor antagonism
    C   NMDA receptor stimulation
    D   Progression of dementia
    E   No response to memantine

47. Administration of clonidine stimulates growth hormone release. What is the mechanism of action?

    A α_1-Adrenoreceptor agonism
    B α_1-Adrenoreceptor antagonism
    C α_2-Adrenoreceptor agonism
    D α_2-Adrenoreceptor antagonism
    E   Imidazoline receptor antagonism

48. A 48-year-old man presented to the accident and emergency department with complaints of inner restlessness, agitation and an inability to sit. He has been taking fluoxetine for the past week for depression. What is the most likely cause for these symptoms?

    A   Blockade of cholinergic receptors in the striatum
    B   Direct dopamine receptor agonism in the striatum
    C   Direct dopamine receptor blockade at the striatum
    D   Indirectly stimulating 5-hydroxytryptamine (5-HT$_{2A}$) receptors which results in excess of dopamine release
    E   Indirectly stimulating 5-HT$_{2A}$ receptors which results in inhibition of dopamine release

49. Ketamine can produce symptoms that are similar to those in schizophrenia. What is the likely mechanism involved?

    A   Blocking NMDA receptors

    B   Glutamate agonist activity
    C   Increasing dopamine activity
    D   Inhibiting glutamate breakdown
    E   Reducing glutamate uptake

50. Which of the following statements about acamprosate is correct?

    A   It inhibits γ-aminobutyric acid neurotransmission
    B   It is a derivative of the amino acid valine
    C   It stimulates glutamate neurotransmission
    D   It stimulates NMDA activity
    E   Its main site of action is the ventral tegmental area

51. If the frequency of the depot antipsychotic injection is every 2 weeks, then how many milligrams of zuclopenthixol decanoate would be approximately equivalent to 40 milligrams of flupenthixol decanoate?

    A   50
    B   100
    C   150
    D   200
    E   250

52. A 42-year-old woman presented with symptoms of stress incontinence. Your consultant asked you to start her on an antidepressant medication. Which of the following would you consider?

    A   Amitriptyline
    B   Duloxetine
    C   Sertraline
    D   Trazodone
    E   Venlafaxine

53. You have discussed the concept of potency of medication in your teachings with medical students. Which of the following selective serotonin reuptake inhibitors is the most potent?

    A   Citalopram
    B   Escitalopram
    C   Fluoxetine
    D   Paroxetine
    E   Sertraline

PSYCHOPHARMACOLOGY: ADVERSE REACTIONS

54. A 46-year-old man with schizophrenia presented to the outpatient clinic with 'fly-catching tongue'. What is the most likely cause of this sign?

    A   Acute dystonic reaction
    B   Catatonic phenomenon
    C   Positive symptoms of schizophrenia
    D   Recent cerebrovascular accident
    E   Tardive dyskinesia

55. Which of the following is most likely due to concomitant use of sodium valproate and lamotrigine?

    A   Lamotrigine levels decrease due to induction of glucuronidation by sodium valproate
    B   Lamotrigine levels increase due to inhibition of glucuronidation by sodium valproate

C   There is no effect on lamotrigine levels
D   Sodium valproate levels increase due to inhibition of glucuronidation by lamotrigine
E   Sodium valproate levels increase due to induction of glucuronidation by lamotrigine

56. Which of the following drugs is least likely to precipitate closed-angle glaucoma?

A   Clozapine
B   Imipramine
C   Lithium
D   Olanzapine
E   Selective serotonin reuptake inhibitors

57. Which of the following is least likely to cause sexual dysfunction?

A   Bupropion
B   Citalopram
C   Imipramine
D   Trazodone
E   Venlafaxine

58. Which of the following antidepressants is recommended in patients who had antidepressant-induced hyperprolactinaemia?

A   Duloxetine
B   Fluoxetine
C   Mirtazapine
D   Paroxetine
E   Venlafaxine

59. A 40-year-old woman with a diagnosis of bipolar affective disorder had four episodes of depression in the past decade and one hypomanic episode 15 years ago. Which of the following drugs is most appropriate as a prophylactic treatment?

A   Carbamazepine
B   Lamotrigine
C   Lithium
D   Olanzapine
E   Valproate

60. Which of the following is the most appropriate first-line antipsychotic to treat psychosis in Parkinson's disease?

A   Aripiprazole
B   Clozapine
C   Olanzapine
D   Paliperidone
E   Quetiapine

PSYCHOPHARMACOLOGY: DRUG DEPENDENCE

61. You have reviewed a 24-year-old man who has misused multiple substances and presented with psychotic symptoms. He was started on quetiapine. He was later prescribed a drug by the substance misuse service after confirmation that he was abstinent from drugs except heroin. Unfortunately, the patient, on taking the drug, collapsed and died. Which of the following is the most likely drug to have been used?

A   Aripiprazole

B   Lofexidine
C   Methadone
D   Naltrexone
E   Suboxone

62. In alcohol dependence, disulfiram is used for aversion therapy. What is its mechanism of action?

    A   It blocks dopamine β-hydroxylase
    B   It is an alcohol dehydrogenase inhibitor
    C   It is an aldehyde dehydrogenase inhibitor
    D   It is a γ-aminobutyric acid A (GABA-A) agonist
    E   It is a GABA-A-receptor antagonist

PSYCHOPHARMACOLOGY: NEW DRUGS

63. Which of the following statements is most accurate about novel treatment approaches being studied for schizophrenia?

    A   Memantine and amantadine are hypothesised to be an option to treat schizophrenia
    B   Metabotrophic postsynaptic glutamate receptors agonists have shown improvements in symptoms of schizophrenia
    C   NMDA antagonists can improve the positive, cognitive and negative symptoms of schizophrenia
    D   NMDA antagonists improve neurons in schizophrenia, so they could be helpful, particularly early in the disease process
    E   NMDA receptors are hyperfunctional in schizophrenia, so glutamate agonists are hypothesised to be helpful to treat it

64. Which of the following statements is most accurate about the novel experimental treatment options for schizophrenia?

    A   D-Cycloserine, a glycine antagonist, has shown some promise for treating schizophrenia
    B   Glycine transporters/Glyt 1 pump inhibitors increase synaptic availability of glycine, and thus reduce NMDA transmission to improve schizophrenia symptoms
    C   LY404039 can reverse phencyclidine (PCP)-induced behavioural changes in animals
    D   Sarcosine is a naturally occurring glycine antagonist that has been shown to improve schizophrenia symptoms
    E   Some amount of dopamine receptor blockade is essential to treat the symptoms of schizophrenia

PSYCHOPHARMACOLOGY: PHARMACOGENETICS

65. Which of the following statements about the implications of COMT genetics is correct?

    A   Met genotype of COMT increases the risk of problems with cognitive performance
    B   Met genotype of COMT predisposes to the risk of schizophrenia
    C   People with Met genotype of COMT have higher dopamine levels
    D   Val genotype of COMT increases the reactivity to life stressors
    E   Val genotype of COMT predisposes to the risk of anxiety disorders

GENETICS: CELLULAR AND MOLECULAR GENETICS

66. In mitotic cell division, which of the following stages of cell division does not involve repetition?

    A   Prophase
    B   Anaphase
    C   Telophase
    D   Interphase
    E   Metaphase

67. 'Knock out' is a technique used in genetics. What is the purpose of this technique?

    A   Linkage analysis
    B   Path analysis
    C   Functional analysis
    D   Genomic analysis
    E   Gene fragmentation analysis

68. Which of the following is consistent with the RNA-splicing enzyme?

    A   Excises large portions of mRNA during transcription
    B   Excises large portions of rRNA during transcription
    C   Excises large portions of tRNA during transcription
    D   Excises large portions of tRNA during translation
    E   Modifies the ends of the RNA molecule

69. What is a possible mechanism to bring about persistent genetic change in response to environmental stressors?

    A   Chromatin remodelling
    B   Nuclear remodelling
    C   Gene regulation
    D   Imprinting Bi genes
    E   Non-epigenetic modification

70. Which of the following has DNA methylation as a critical step?

    A   Chromatin remodelling
    B   Gene expression
    C   Imprinting
    D   Transcription
    E   Translation

71. The chromatids of the homologous chromosome in the metaphase of meiosis exchange segments by breakage. What is this called?

    A   Genetic linkage
    B   Independent assortment
    C   Recombination
    D   Segregation
    E   Synapsis

72. On which of the following is chromosomal analysis usually carried out?

    A   Amniotic fluid
    B   Bone marrow
    C   Red blood cells
    D   Skin
    E   White blood cells

73. What is aneuploidy?

    A   Alteration in the number of sex chromosomes
    B   Alteration in the number of autosomes
    C   Alteration in the number of sex chromosomes or autosomes
    D   Description of the fragile site on a chromosome
    E   Gain of an extra segment of chromosome

74. Which of the following about robertsonian translocation is correct?

    A   Exchange of segment between two different pairs of chromosomes
    B   Fusion of two chromosomes at their centromere
    C   Translocation of a segment of one chromosome on a fragile site to another chromosome
    D   When segment of a chromosome included twice over
    E   When segment of chromosome detached and then reattached in opposite orientation

75. Which of the following shows anticipation?

    A   Dynamic mutation
    B   Frame-shift mutation
    C   Genomic imprinting
    D   Mitochondrial mutation
    E   Substitution mutation

76. What defect is seen in disorders of 'imprinting' such as Prader–Willi syndrome and Angelman's syndrome?

    A   DNA methylation
    B   Pleiotropy
    C   Reverse transcriptase
    D   RNA coding
    E   Transcription factors

77. What does the term 'horizontal inheritance' in genetics mean?

    A   Transmission of disease from mother to child
    B   Transmission of disease from father to child
    C   The phenomenon in which affected individuals are found in every generation
    D   The phenomenon in which affected individuals are seen every second generation
    E   No case occurring in previous generation, but the disease manifesting in children of next generation

GENETICS: BEHAVIOURAL GENETICS

78. Gene mapping helps to locate and identify genes in psychiatric disorders. What is the most widely used genetic marker for gene mapping?

    A   Microsatellites
    B   Restriction fragment length polymorphism
    C   Short tandem repeats
    D   Single nucleotide polymorphism
    E   Variable number tandem repeats

79. The fact that 'high levels of licking and grooming in early life of rat pups by mothers alter brain glucocorticoid expression and stress sensitivity in offspring' is an example of gene regulation. Which of the following is involved in this process?

    A   Inherited DNA or RNA

     B   Endogenous factors
     C   Environmental factors by biological mechanism
     D   Epigenetics
     E   Genetic linkage

80. What do we call the study of diseases in families when co-segregation of the disease and a set of genetic markers are investigated?

     A   Gene mapping
     B   Genetic algorithm
     C   Genetic association
     D   Genetic coding
     E   Genetic linkage

81. Which of the following statements about the recombinant fraction is correct?

     A   It is expressed in centimorgans
     B   It is the most important parameter involved in gene mapping
     C   It is the proportion of cross-over that occurs in metaphase of mitosis
     D   It is the total number of recombinants multiplied by number of off-springs
     E   It is zero when the two loci are very close together

82. In linkage analysis, what logarithm of the odd (LOD) score is accepted by convention to signify the linkage that has been detected?

     A   −2
     B   −1
     C   1
     D   2
     E   3

GENETICS: ENDOPHENOTYPES

83. Which of the following statements best describes the Hardy–Weinberg equilibrium?

     A   Genetic variation in a population will remain constant from one generation to the next in the absence of disturbing factors
     B   In a population, both genotype and allelic frequencies keep changing
     C   The phenotype and allelic frequencies in a population are not in equilibrium
     D   There is a continuous change of phenotypes in a population from one generation to the next
     E   There is a continuous change of genes in a population from one generation to the next

84. A 38-year-old white man migrated to the USA and started a new relationship with an Asian woman. They have two children. How are the genetic changes that occur in his children best described?

     A   Gene drift
     B   Gene flow
     C   Genetic recombination
     D   Independent assortment
     E   Random mating

85. To which of the following genes is P50 suppression linked?

     A   Cannabinoid receptor-1 gene
     B   Dopamine receptor-1 gene

C   Histamine receptor gene
D   Nicotinic receptor gene
E   Serotonin receptor gene

GENETICS: GENETIC EPIDEMIOLOGY

86. You are assessing a 14-year-old boy with a family history suggestive of both parents having schizophrenia. What are the chances of this boy developing schizophrenia?

A   5%
B   10%
C   30%
D   50%
E   85%

87. Which of the following statements about twin studies in schizophrenia is correct?

A   Dizygotic (DZ) probandwise concordance rate is around 24%
B   More than four-fifths of the variance in causes of schizophrenia are genetically determined
C   Monozygotic (MZ) probandwise concordance rate is around 66%
D   Probandwise concordance rate is defined as the percentage of probands who have an affected sibling whether or not a twin
E   Probandwise concordance rates are the same using the ICD-10 and DSM-IV criteria

88. Which of the following statements about genetics in eating disorders is correct?

A   Among female siblings of patients with established anorexia nervosa (AN), 5–10% of them have the condition compared with 0.5–1.0% found in the general population of the same age
B   Concordance rate for AN in DZ twins is 15%
C   Concordance rate for AN in MZ twins is 40%
D   Inherited liability to AN does not involve relevant personality traits such as perfectionism and obsessionality
E   There is no association between eating disorders and mood disorders

89. Which of the following statements about family and twin studies in unipolar depression and bipolar affective disorder is correct?

A   In unipolar depression, the concordance rate is 46% in MZ and 20% in DZ twins
B   Overall, the genetic influence in bipolar affective disorder is less than in unipolar depression
C   Relatives of bipolar probands have an increased risk of schizoaffective disorder and bipolar affective disorder, but not unipolar depression
D   Relatives of patients with unipolar depression have an increased risk of bipolar or schizoaffective disorder
E   The concordance rate for mood disorders in the MZ co-twin of a proband with bipolar affective disorder is between 60 and 70%, and for DZ twins the rate is about 40%

GENETICS: GENE–ENVIRONMENT INTERACTION

90. In twin studies focusing on the role of genetic and environmental factors in adolescent alcohol misuse, genetic factors played a large role. Where did these adolescents live?

A   Equal role in both urban and rural areas
B   Rural areas

   C   Suburban areas
   D   Urban areas
   E   Villages

91. Which of the following statements about twin studies investigating gene–environment interactions in generalised anxiety disorder (GAD) and major depression (MD) is correct?

   A   Common familial environment is an aetiological factor in both GAD and MD
   B   Genes that influenced lifetime risk for GAD and MD are not shared between two disorders
   C   Stressful life events that involve a loss lead to GAD
   D   Stressful life events that involve danger lead to MD
   E   Stressful life events that involve a threat lead to GAD

92. A 16-year-old boy carried genes that make him interact less with others. He was shy and isolated himself. This led to bullying in school and depression. What is this process of genetic factors influencing the environment that a person chooses called?

   A   Gene–environment correlation
   B   Gene–environment adaptation
   C   Gene–environment influence
   D   Gene–environment interaction
   E   Gene–environment manipulation

93. A 74-year-old man had genetic testing for insurance purposes and was found to have the ε4 allele. He had intact cognitive functions. In this case, what is the ε4 gene called?

   A   Association gene
   B   Causative gene
   C   Risk gene
   D   Susceptibility gene
   E   Vulnerability gene

94. A 70-year-old white man had genetic testing for insurance purposes. He has intact cognitive functions. In which of the following situations is he at maximum risk of developing Alzheimer's disease?

   A   A positive family history of Alzheimer's disease
   B   Presence of ε2/ε3 allele
   C   Past history of head injury
   D   Presence of one ε4 allele
   E   Presence of one ε4 allele and past history of head injury

EPIDEMIOLOGY: SURVEYS ACROSS THE LIFESPAN

95. What is the prevalence rate of autism in patients with learning disability/intellectual disability?

   A   3%
   B   5%
   C   7%
   D   9%
   E   10%

96. What is the prevalence of schizophrenia in people with learning disability/intellectual disability?

   A   1%
   B   2%

C   3%
D   4%
E   5%

97. What is the prevalence of borderline personality disorder in community surveys?

A   0.1
B   0.4
C   0.6
D   0.7
E   4.0

98. How many schoolchildren are on average affected by developmental dyslexia (specific reading difficulty) in English-speaking countries?

A   0.4–0.8%
B   1–3%
C   3–6%
D   6–8%
E   8–10%

99. What is the lifetime prevalence rate of self-harm in youths identifying themselves with the Goth subculture?

A   13%
B   25%
C   33%
D   47%
E   53%

100. What is the lifetime suicide risk in patients with schizophrenia?

A   4–5%
B   8–10%
C   10–13%
D   13–15%
E   15–20%

101. What is the estimated prevalence rate for anorexia nervosa?

A   0.1%
B   0.2%
C   0.3%
D   0.4%
E   0.5%

102. What is the incidence rate of bulimia nervosa per 100,000 people per year?

A   8
B   10
C   13
D   15
E   17

103. What is the prevalence of depression in the > 65 year age group in men and women combined?

A   8%
B   10%

C   12%
D   14%
E   16%

104. Approximately how many residents in the UK might have a personality disorder?

A   1 in 5
B   1 in 10
C   1 in 15
D   1 in 20
E   1 in 25

105. Which of the following is consistent with vascular dementia?

A   Its frequency has shown a reduction in recent studies in older individuals
B   Its incidence is not affected by stroke or cerebrovascular disorders
C   It is more prevalent in men than in women
D   It is the third commonest cause of dementia
E   Its prevalence has been static over a period of 10 years from age 60 years

106. Which of the following statements about schizophrenia is correct?

A   Association of schizophrenia is seen with maternal age in patients with a family history of schizophrenia.
B   Association of schizophrenia is seen with maternal age in patients with no family history of schizophrenia.
C   Association of schizophrenia is seen with parental age in patients with a family history of schizophrenia.
D   Association of schizophrenia is seen with paternal age in patients with no family history of schizophrenia.
E   Association of schizophrenia is seen with both paternal and maternal age in patients with a family history of schizophrenia.

107. Which of the following statements about the outcomes of schizophrenia, schizoaffective and affective disorders is correct?

A   Schizophrenia has a better outcome than schizoaffective but poorer than affective disorders
B   Schizoaffective disorder has a better outcome than schizophrenia but poorer than affective disorders
C   Affective disorders have a better outcome than schizoaffective disorder but poorer than schizophrenia
D   Schizophrenia has a better outcome than schizoaffective and affective disorders
E   Affective disorders have a better outcome than schizoaffective disorder or schizophrenia

108. The suicide rate per 100,000 in women was found to be highest in one of the countries than what was expected from the study by the World Health Organization (WHO 2003). Which country was it?

A   Belarus
B   China
C   Japan
D   Lithuania
E   Sri Lanka

109. In which age group was the suicide rate the highest by sex and age in the UK from 2000 to 2009?

A   15- to 44-year-old females
B   15- to 44-year-old males
C   45- to 74-year-old females

D   45- to 74-year-old males
E   75+ males/females

110. The global WHO distribution (2000) of suicide rate per 100,000 by age and gender reveals the maximum suicide rate in both males and females. In what age group does this occur?

A   15–24 years
B   25–34 years
C   55–64 years
D   65–74 years
E   75+ years

EPIDEMIOLOGY: MEASURES

111. A recent study identified that, in a defined population of 8 million people, there were 30,000 live-born babies. Of these, 120 died before they could see their first birthday and 150 before they turned 5. What is infant mortality rate in this population?

A   1
B   3
C   4
D   5
E   6

112. Which of the following rating scales is often used in long-term outcome studies of eating disorders?

A   Bech–Rafaelsen rating scale
B   Conners' rating scale
C   Morgan–Russell assessment schedule
D   Vanderbilt's assessment scale
E   Wender's Utah rating scale

113. In a 6-year follow-up study, of 100 people who used cannabis, 20 developed schizophrenia. This was compared with 100 people who did not use cannabis among whom 5 developed schizophrenia. What is the odds ratio?

A   0.2
B   0.4
C   4
D   5
E   6

114. Which of the following rating scales is generally administered by trained non-clinicians?

A   Diagnostic interview schedule
B   Global assessment of functioning scale
C   Positive and negative symptoms scale
D   Schedule for assessment in neuropsychiatry
E   Structured clinical interview for the DSM-IV

115. Which of the following about case registry is correct?

A   Most of the clinical data is available
B   Independent of other registers
C   Individually based
D   Non-cumulative
E   Prospective

116. Which of the following rating scales was used in National Comorbidity Survey conducted in 1990–1992?

    A   Composite international diagnostic interview
    B   Diagnostic interview schedule
    C   Global assessment of functioning scale
    D   Present state examination
    E   Structured clinical interview for the DSM-IV

117. Which of the following statements about Beck's depression inventory is correct?

    A   It can be graded into cognitive and somatic subscales
    B   It contains 25 questions
    C   It doesn't correlate well with the HAM-D score
    D   It is a clinician-administered scale
    E   It measures the nature of depression

A new diagnostic test was administered in a population of 10000. The results showed true positive = 35, false positive = 10, true negative = 9940 and false negative = 15. **Use this data for questions 119–123.**

118. What is the sensitivity of the new test?

    A $(35/50) \times 100$
    B $(35/45) \times 100$
    C $(9940/9950) \times 100$
    D $(10/45) \times 100$
    E $(10/50) \times 100$

119. In the example above, what is the specificity of the test?

    A $(35/50) \times 100$
    B $(35/45) \times 100$
    C $(9940/9950) \times 100$
    D $(10/45) \times 100$
    E $(10/50) \times 100$

120. In the example above, what is the prevalence?

    A $(35/50) \times 100$
    B $(35/45) \times 100$
    C $(9940/9950) \times 100$
    D $(10/45) \times 100$
    E $50/10000$

121. In the example above, what is the positive predictive value?

    A $(35/50) \times 100$
    B $(35/45) \times 100$
    C $(9940/9950) \times 100$
    D $(10/45) \times 100$
    E $(10/50) \times 100$

122. In the example above, what is the negative predictive value?

    A $(35/50) \times 100$
    B $(35/45) \times 100$
    C $(9940/9950) \times 100$
    D $(10/45) \times 100$
    E $(10/50) \times 100$

ADVANCED PSYCHOLOGICAL PROCESSES AND TREATMENTS: PERSONALITY AND PERSONALITY DISORDER

123. Which of the following is one of Cloninger's temperamental dimensions of personality?

    A   Cooperativeness
    B   Novelty aversion
    C   Reward dependence
    D   Self-directedness
    E   Self-transcendence

124. Which of the following statements is most accurate about antisocial personality disorder?

    A   Comorbidity with axis I disorders is uncommon
    B   Interventions focusing on improving the parent–child attachment can have benefits for primary schoolchildren who are at risk of developing conduct disorders
    C   Therapeutic community approach is helpful in reducing reoffending after release in offenders with drug and alcohol misuse.
    D   There is very limited research establishing the efficacy of cognitive–behavioural therapy in reducing reoffending
    E   There is very limited research establishing the efficacy of a functional family to benefit treatment of adolescents with conduct disorders

125. Which of the following statements about brief psychological interventions used in patients with borderline personality disorder is correct?

    A   Manually assisted cognitive therapy is a type of brief psychological intervention
    B   They are brief but high-intensity interventions
    C   They are delivered for about 6–9 months
    D   They have been found to be significantly more cost-effective than usual treatment
    E   There is a good evidence base for such interventions in borderline patients

126. Which of the following statements about evidence-based psychological therapies in patients with borderline personality disorder is correct?

    A   Individual psychotherapy has been found to be superior to cognitive–behavioural therapy (CBT)
    B   Non-randomized controlled trial (RCT) evidence suggests that individual psychological therapies are well accepted by patients and show positive outcomes
    C   Significant benefits of treatment have been seen by CBT compared with usual treatment
    D   There is a good RCT evidence base for some of the individual psychological interventions
    E   There is strong evidence to suggest that cognitive–analytical therapy (CAT) in young people improves their general functioning and reduces self-harm

127. Which of the following statements about dialectical behavioural therapy (DBT) for patients with borderline personality disorder is correct?

    A   'Coaching' is the weekly supervision that the therapist has with the supervisor
    B   Dialectical strategies encompass aspects of both acceptance and change
    C   It was first developed by Linehan for men who self-harm
    D   It has five stages in the treatment process
    E   Weekly individual therapies are avoided while DBT is being delivered

128. Which of the following statements about therapeutic communities is correct?

    A   Behavioural interventions are rarely included as part of community meetings
    B   Medication is prohibited for personality disorders in some therapeutic communities

C   Most communities operate a rolling programme of 3–6 months
D   The ultimate aim of a therapeutic community is to treat the disorder
E   They are usually monthly residential units

129. Which of the following statements about metallisation-based therapy (MBT) for borderline personality disorder patients is correct?

A   Although it helps reduce suicide attempts, it does not affect depressive symptoms
B   It is not suitable for outpatient settings
C   It is a form of CBT
D   It was devised by Bateman and Fonagy in 2004
E   When combined with partial hospitalisation, it is delivered for a maximum of 12 months

ADVANCED PSYCHOLOGICAL PROCESSES AND TREATMENTS: DEVELOPMENTAL PSYCHOPATHOLOGY (INCLUDING TEMPERAMENT)

130. Which of the following is a preferred parenting style?

A   Authoritarian
B   Authoritative
C   Enmeshed
D   Neglectful
E   Permissive

131. Which of the following statements about the Oedipus complex is correct?

A   Concept of Oedipus complex was first discussed by Anna Freud
B   It starts from the age of 2 years
C   The boy develops anger towards his father and wishes to castrate him (father)
D   The boy acquires super-ego through repression of his feelings towards the love object
E   To resolve the complex, the boy represses his desires for his mother and his hostile feelings for his father

132. According to Sigmund Freud, which of the following is a part of the structural model of the mind?

A   Conscious
B   Ego
C   Oedipus
D   Preconscious
E   Unconscious

133. According to Sigmund Freud, which area of the structural model extends through all three topographical domains?

A   Ego
B   Conscious
C   Id
D   Super-ego
E   Unconscious

134. Which of the following is a kleinian stage of human development?

A   Anal
B   Anima
C   Phallic

D   Paranoid schizoid position
E   Transitional zone

135. According to Winnicott, which term describes the concept of a soft toy that buffers against loss and gets invested with a primary object's qualities?

A   Collective unconscious
B   Good-enough mother
C   Individuation
D   Multiple self-organisation
E   Transitional object

136. Which of the following figures in developmental psychopathology was central to the school of object relations theory?

A   Burrhus Frederic Skinner
B   Carl Gustav Jung
C   Carl Rogers
D   Melanie Klein
E   Sigmund Freud

137. According to Melanie Klein which of the following developmental stages is considered to be castration of the infant?

A   Crawling
B   Breastfeeding
C   Imperfect mother
D   Toilet training
E   Weaning

138. Which of the following statements about the assessment of attachment in adults is correct?

A   Adler devised the adult attachment interview
B   Attachment can be assessed only in psychiatric patients
C   Interview measures may be better than self-report measures
D   The adult attachment interview does not require training
E   Self-report measures should not be used because they do not have validity

139. Which of the following statements about investigator-based diagnostic interview measures in psychiatry is correct?

A   Behaviours are rated by the patient as to whether or not the phenomenon is present
B   They do not take too much time to conduct
C   Structure resides in the investigator's conceptualisation of the phenomenon being studied
D   There is no emphasis on eliciting descriptions of behaviours
E   Usually no training is required

140. Which of the following statements about respondent-based diagnostic interviews is correct?

A   Questions can be rephrased
B   Lay people can deliver these interviews
C   They require training
D   They are used in randomized controlled trials of new psychotropic drugs
E   It takes time to deliver these interviews

141. Which of the following statements about diagnosis, based on lists of criteria in child psychiatry, is correct?

A   Children who meet the criteria really have the problem
B   Children with significant impairment meet the criteria

    C   Labels can be helpful
    D   Labelling does not lead to stigma
    E   There is no overlap between different diagnoses

142. Which of the following statements about the relationship between a parent and a child is correct?

    A   It can be improved by teaching skills to the parent
    B   It is regulated by the principles of classic conditioning
    C   It involves only the efforts of a parent to establish the relationship
    D   It is the only attachment relationship formed by a child
    E   It is unaffected by parental mental illness

143. Which of the following statements about the assessment of patients in a family context is correct?

    A   It is based on practical considerations
    B   It reduces the importance of individual diagnosis
    C   It reduces the likelihood of detecting a psychiatric disorder
    D   It reduces the need for a mental state examination
    E   It requires all family members to be seen together

ADVANCED PSYCHOLOGICAL PROCESSES AND TREATMENTS: THERAPY MODELS, METHODS, PROCESSES AND OUTCOMES

144. Which of the following techniques is a key technique used in DBT?

    A   Distress tolerance
    B   Externalising the problem
    C   Habit reversal
    D   Restricted role repertoire
    E   Thought stopping

145. Which of the following is a stage according to Prochaska and DiClemente's model of motivational interview?

    A   Abstinence
    B   Contemplation
    C   Projection
    D   Resolution
    E   Stagnation

146. Which of the following is a cognitive distortion?

    A   Metaphor
    B   Selective abstraction
    C   Splitting
    D   Triangulation
    E   Trap

147. In which of the following disorders has systemic therapy been shown to be effective?

    A   Adult personality disorders
    B   Anxiety disorders

C   Childhood asthma
D   Obsessive–compulsive disorder
E   Trauma-related disorder

148. Which of the following defence mechanisms is considered to be of immature type?

A   Humour
B   Intellectualisation
C   Inhibition
D   Regression
E   Sexualisation

149. A 50-year-old man was diagnosed with cancer. When told about the diagnosis, he responded by saying that he had a good life and that may be it was his 'time'. Which defence mechanism is being displayed?

A   Acting out
B   Altruism
C   Dissociation
D   Rationalisation
E   Repression

150. Which of the following statements about conditioning is correct?

A   Classic conditioning is also known as instrumental conditioning
B   Law of effect was suggested by Albert Ellis
C   Learning takes longer in direct learning than vicarious reinforcement
D   Operant conditioning is also known as pavlovian conditioning
E   Phobias are maintained by operant conditioning

151. Which of the following is the most appropriate psychological intervention for mild alcohol dependence?

A   Cognitive-behaviour therapy
B   Family therapy
C   Group therapy
D   Interpersonal therapy
E   Psychodynamic psychotherapy

152. Which of the following statements about psychological interventions in children and young people who abuse alcohol is correct?

A   Brief strategic family therapy should be offered twice weekly for a month to support the family
B   Functional family therapy helps to focus on parents' wellbeing and parenting skills
C   Functional family therapy should be conducted over 6–9 months
D   Multidimensional family therapy should consist of 12–15 sessions
E   Multidimensional family therapy should be offered over 24–30 weeks

ADVANCED PSYCHOLOGICAL PROCESSES AND TREATMENTS: PSYCHOSOCIAL INFLUENCES

153. Who was first to link the development of psychopathy to parental neglect?

A   Johnson
B   Kohut

C   Marshall and Cook
D   McCord and McCord
E   Ploman and Bergmann

154. Which of the following statements about early life adversity is correct?

A   Boys show more deprivation features than girls
B   Deprivation leads to non-formation of attachment
C   Loving care-giving leads to privation
D   Privation is more common than deprivation
E   Privation occurs after formation of attachment

Answers: MCQs

1. D Paresis of face and arm

The medial striate artery, also known as the recurrent artery of Heubner, is the largest perforating branch of the anterior cerebral artery. An occlusion in the unilateral medial striate artery gives rise to contralateral paresis of the face and arm, dysarthria and hemichorea. An occlusion of the bilateral medial striate artery results in akinetic mutism. Ideomotor apraxia is caused by an occlusion in the pericallosal branch of the anterior cerebral artery. Apathy with some memory loss is caused by an occlusion in the orbitofrontal polar branch of the anterior cerebral artery occlusion. Tactile anomia is an inability to recognise an object when presented by touch in the absence of aphasic anomia. It can occur due to a lesion in the corpus callosum resulting in a disconnection between the tactile and language areas of the brain.

2. A Dysarthria–clumsy hand syndrome

The internal capsule is divided into three components such as the anterior limb, genu and posterior limb. There are five classical lacunar syndromes described in the literature with characteristics signs. Lacunar infarct in the genu of internal capsules gives rise to dysarthria, clumsiness of one hand with or without central facial paralysis, dysphasia and tongue deviation, also known as dysarthria–clumsy hand syndrome. Pure motor stroke is the commonest type of lacunar infarct. It occurs due to an infarct in the posterior limb of the internal capsule and presents with contralateral hemiparesis, facial weakness with or without dysarthria, and bilateral pure motor stroke. Lacunar infarcts in the ventral posterior nucleus of the thalamus give rise to a pure sensory syndrome with or without sensory ataxia. Lacunar infarcts in either the anterior or the posterior internal capsule can also lead to sensorimotor stroke or ataxic hemiparesis.

3. A Body-image formation

Agnosis is an abnormality in the perception of sensation despite a normal sensory pathway. Anosognosia, which is unawareness of weakness of the affected side, is associated with a non-dominant parietal lobe lesion. Non-dominant parietal and occipital lesions are linked with visual and body perception. Other options mentioned in the question occur because of a lesion in the dominant hemisphere.

4. E Temporal lobe

A lesion in the middle and inferior temporal gyrus is associated with memory loss, déjà-vu, jamais-vu and difficulties in learning. A lesion in the auditory cortex of the temporal lobe is associated with cortical deafness, Wernicke's aphasia (dominant side) and tinnitus. A lesion involving the limbic part of the temporal lobe results in aggressive behaviour, inability to learn new memory and olfactory hallucination. A lesion in the optic radiation is associated with upper homonymous quadrantanopia.

5. D Non-dominant parietal lobe

A lesion in the non-dominant parietal lobe can cause difficulty in calculation, spatial and perceptual disorientation, hemispatial neglect, anosognosia, dyspraxia and agnosia. A lesion in the dominant parietal lobe can cause receptive aphasia, Gerstmann's syndrome and dyslexia. Balint's syndrome is associated with a bilateral parietal lobe lesion.

6. A Amygdaloid nucleus

The limbic lobe is an arrangement of cortical structures around the diencephalon. It consists of cortical areas and nuclei. The cortical areas include cingulate gyrus, parahippocampal gyrus and subcallosal gyrus, whereas nuclei include the amygdaloid nucleus and septal nucleus.

7. B Corpus striatum

Basal ganglia are a collection of nuclei located at the base of the forebrain. It consists of the corpus striatum, globus pallidus, substantia nigra, nucleus accumbens and subthalamic nuclei. The corpus striatum is the largest of all the components and is further subdivided into the caudate nucleus and putamen. The dentate nucleus is located in the cerebellar hemisphere. The amygdaloid nucleus, septal nucleus and cingulate gyrus are components of the limbic system.

8. D Vagus nerve

The intrinsic muscles of the larynx and constrictor muscles of the pharynx are supplied by the motor fibres of the vagus nerve (cranial nerve X). The vestibulocochlear nerve (cranial nerve VIII) supplies sensory fibres to the internal ear. The spinal accessory nerve (cranial nerve XI) supplies trapezius and sternocleidomastoid. The hypoglossal nerve (cranial nerve XII) supplies motor fibres to intrinsic muscles of the tongue, styloglossus, hyoglossus and genioglossus. The trochlear nerve (cranial nerve IV) supplies the superior oblique muscle in the eyes.

9. C Neural plates

The entire nervous system originates from the neural plate, which is an ectodermal thickening in the floor of the amniotic sac. During the third week after fertilisation, the plate forms paired neural folds that unite to create the neural tube and canal. The open ends of the tube, which are known as neuropores, are closed off before the end of the fourth week. The process of formation of the neural tube from the ectoderm is called neurulation.

10. D Fourth week

The neural tube is the precursor of the brain and spinal cord. The formation of the neural tube begins in the third week of gestation and is completed by the middle of the fourth week. The neural tube develops by primary and secondary neurulation. It develops into the prosencephalon, mesencephalon, rhombencephalon and spinal cord.

11. B Mesencephalon

During the development of an organism, the midline neural tube differentiates into the prosencephalon, telencephalon, diencephalon, and rhombencephalon. The diencephalon differentiates into the thalamus, subthalamus, hypothalamus and epithalamus. The mesencephalon differentiates into tectum, basis pedunculi and tegmentum.

12. E Telencephalon

The prosencephalon differentiates into the telencephalon, which in turn gives rise to the cerebral hemispheres and differentiates into the pallidum, corpus striatum, medullary centre and rhinencephalon. The rhombencephalon differentiates into the metencephalon which further differentiates into the pons, oral part of the medulla and cerebellum. The mylencephalon further differentiates into the caudal part of the medulla oblongata.

13. D Rhombencephalon

This is also known as the hindbrain. It consists of the pons, medulla and cerebellum. The rhombencephalon forms the myelencephalon, which forms the medulla oblongata, and the metencephalon, which forms the pons and cerebellum. The neural tube closure possibly begins at the caudal end of the rhombencephalon.

14. C Reactive astrocytosis

The histolopathological changes that are seen in Pick's disease include pick bodies, neuronal loss and reactive astrocytosis. The macroscopic changes seen in Pick's disease are selective and asymmetrical atrophy of the anterior frontal and temporal lobes, knife blade gyri and ventricular enlargement. The macroscopic changes that are seen in Alzheimer's disease include global brain atrophy, ventricular enlargement and sulcus widening. These changes are mostly seen in the frontal and temporal lobes.

15. B Changes including infarction and ischaemia

The histolopathological changes that are seen in multi-infarct dementia include signs of infarction and ischaemia. The macroscopic changes seen in multi-infarct dementia are multiple cerebral infarcts, local and general brain atrophy, ventricular enlargement and arteriosclerotic changes in the major arteries. Sulci widening is mainly seen in Alzheimer's dementia.

16. A Alzheimer's disease

Patients who are diagnosed with Alzheimer's disease show both tau and β-amyloid inclusions and deposits. Hence, it can be classified as both a tauopathy and an amyloidopathy.

Table 3.1 Dementia–amyloidopathy and tauopathy	
Amyloidopathy–presence of β-amyloid plaques	Tauopathy–presence of tau inclusions
Sporadic Alzheimer's disease	Pick's disease
Familial Alzheimer's disease	Progressive supranuclear palsy
Down's syndrome (trisomy 21)	Frontotemporal dementia with parkinsonism associated with chromosome 17
Amyloid angiopathy	Corticobasal degeneration

17. D Prion deposition

Consortium criteria (Consortium to establish a registry for Alzheimer's disease [CERAD]) are used for the evaluation and diagnosis of patients with Alzheimer's disease. It has been translated into several languages including English and used worldwide. The criteria were set by correlating clinical progression with histopathological findings on postmortem examination of the brain of patients who had Alzheimer's dementia. The neuropathological criteria are assessment of amyloid plaque deposition, pallor of the substantia nigra, ventricular dilatation, state of the vessels, lacunar or large infarcts, neurofibrillary tangles and Lewy bodies. The amyloid plaque density is assessed in various cortical areas such as the hippocampus, entorhinal cortex and midbrain.

18. D Tuberous sclerosis

The clinical and pathological features of tuberous sclerosis include a shagreen patch, subungual angiofibroma, glial nodules in the cortex and adjacent to the ventricles, rhabdomyoma of the heart, learning disability and epilepsy. It is a rare genetic disease caused by a mutation of genes such as *TSC1* and *TSC2*. It results in non-malignant tumours in the brain, kidney, eyes, lungs, heart and skin. Ataxia telangiectasia is a rare disorder that presents with telangiectasia of the skin and conjunctiva, progressive ataxia from childhood, IgA deficiency and thymic hypoplasia. Sturge–Weber syndrome consists of a strawberry naevus/port wine stain on the face, angiomatous malformation of meningeal vessels with calcification, along with learning disability and epilepsy. Von Hippel–Lindau disease is a rare disorder and presents with vascular malformation of the retina, haemangioblastoma, pancreatic, adrenal and renal cysts, and tumour. Von Recklinghausen's neurofibromatosis presents with cutaneous neurofibromas including plexiform-type Lisch nodules in the iris, learning disability and intracranial tumours.

19. A Gliomas

The most common cerebral tumours are gliomas which are derived from glial cells and their precursors. These tumours include astrocytomas, oligodendrocytomas and ependymomas. The following cerebral tumours are arranged in relative frequency of occurrence: gliomas, metastases, meningeal tumours, pituitary adenomas, neurilemmomas, haemangioblastomas and medulloblastomas.

20. B 3–5

A normal sleep is characterised by three to five sleep cycles per night. It is broadly divided into two types: rapid eye movement (REM) and non-rapid eye movement (NREM) sleep types. An adult usually spends 20–25% of total sleep time in REM sleep. The usual order of the sleep cycle is NREM stage 1, NREM stage 2, NREM stage 3, NREM stage 2 and REM. The REM sleep is also known as paradoxical sleep and NREM sleep as slow-wake sleep.

21. A Aα

The conduction velocity of an electrochemical signal in a nerve depends upon several factors such as axon diameter, myelination, temperature and internal resistance in the axon. Nerve fibres are largely classified as motor, sensory, preganglionic or postganglionic fibres. According to the Erlanger/Gasser classification, the nerve conduction velocity of different fibres such as Aα, Aβ, Aγ, Aδ, B and C is 70–120, 30–70, 15–30, 12–30, 3–15 and 0.5 m/s, respectively.

22. C GABA-B

The major neurotransmitter system of the nervous system is divided into fast, moderate and slow types. The fast transmitters are linked with the ion channel with a speed of 3–10 m/s, moderate transmitters are linked with the second messenger system with a speed of 10–100 m/s, and slow transmitters are linked with the peptides with a speed of 100 m/s and over. GABA-B receptors are associated with moderate second messenger transmitters. Receptors such as α-amino-3-hydroxy-5-methyl-4-isoxazolepropionic acid (AMPA), GABA-A, kainate, glycine, nicotine, 5-hydroxytryptamine 3, and NMDA are linked with fast ion channels that have a speed of 3–10 m/s.

23. D Histamines (H_1, H_2 and H_3)

There are two major types of receptors: ionotropic and metabotropic receptors. Neurotransmitters that activate metabotropic receptors include glutamate–mGluRs, GABA-B, acetylcholine (muscarinic), and dopamine: D_1/D_2, serotonin: $5\text{-}HT_1/5\text{-}HT_2$, noradrenaline, histamine $H_1/H_2/H_3$, all types of neuropeptides and adenosine. Neurotransmitters that activate ionotropic receptors include glutamate, AMPA-K, GABA-A, acetylcholine, nicotine and glycine, serotonin (or $5\text{-}HT_3$) and purines. Metabotropic receptors, once activated, act indirectly, whereas ionotropic receptors act directly by opening ion channels.

24. C Clathrin

In the transmitter transport system and vesicle recycling, the actin protein brings vesicles into contact with the presynaptic membrane. Synaptophysin proteins create the membrane fusion pore. Calmodulin protein expels the vesicle contents into the synaptic cleft. Dynamin protein pinches the neck of the developing vesicles to complete its separation. Clathrin protein withdraws the vesicle membrane from the synaptic cleft.

25. C Expels vesicle content into the synaptic cleft

In the transmitter transport system and vesicle recycling, the actin protein brings vesicles into contact with the presynaptic membrane. Synaptophysin protein creates the membrane fusion pore. Calmodulin protein expels vesicle contents into the synaptic cleft. Dynamin protein pinches the neck of the developing vesicles to complete its separation. Clathrin protein withdraws the vesicle membrane from the synaptic cleft.

26. D III

There are two main classifications for nerve fibres such as Erlanger/Gasser and Lloyd Hunt classification systems. In the Lloyd Hunt classification system, only the sensory fibres are classified as I, II, III and IV fibres. The fibres Ia, Ib, II, III and IV innervate muscle spindle afferents, tendon organs, cutaneous mechanoreceptors, deep pressure sensors in muscle and unmyelinated pain fibres, respectively. In the Erlanger/Gasser classification system, both motor and sensory fibres are classified as A, B and C fibres.

27. C II

As per the Lloyd Hunt classification system, the nerves are classified as Ia, Ib, II, III and IV. The conduction velocity of I, II, III and IV nerve fibres is 70–120 m/s, 25–70 m/s, 10–25 m/s and 1 m/s, respectively.

28. A Antidiuretic hormone

Hormones that are secreted from the posterior pituitary gland are the antidiuretic hormone or vasopressin and oxytocin. Hormones that are secreted from the anterior pituitary are growth hormone (somatotrophin), thyroid-stimulating hormone (thyrotrophin), adrenocorticotrophin and β-endorphin (corticotrophin), prolactin (lactotrophin), luteinising and follicular-stimulating hormones (gonadotrophins) and melanocyte-stimulating hormone (melanotrophins).

29. E Dopamine β-hydroxylase

Dopamine is a precursor of neurotransmitters such as noradrenaline and adrenaline. It is converted to noradrenaline by dopamine β-hydroxylase. Acetyl-coenzyme A facilitates the production of acetylcholine from choline. Alcohol dehydrogenase and aldehyde dehydrogenase enzymes are responsible for the disulfiram reaction.

30. E Catechol-*O*-methyltransferase

Monoamines are transported across the cells by dopamine, serotonin and noradrenaline transporters in the outer cell membrane and across the intracellular vesicles by vesicle monoamine transporter. The enzyme that is responsible for the degradation of monoamines in the synapse is catechol-*O*-methyltransferase (COMT) and in the presynaptic neuron vesicles it is monoamine oxidase.

31. C L-tyrosine

As far as precursors are concerned choline and acetyl-coenzyme A are precursors of acetylcholine, and L-tyrosine, L-dopa and dopamine are precursors of noradrenaline. L-Tryptophan is the precursor of serotonin. L-Tyrosine and L-dopa are precursors of dopamine and histidine is the precursor of histamine.

32. E Synthesised from L-tyrosine

L-Tyrosine is the precursor of catecholamines such as adrenaline, noradrenaline and dopamine. L-Tyrosine is first converted to L-dopa by hydroxylation and then to dopamine by decarboxylation. Therefore, L-dopa is the immediate precursor of dopamine. Once formed, dopamine is stored in the presynaptic complex. It is converted to noradrenaline by β-hydroxylation and hence is the immediate precursor of noradrenaline. It is degraded by COMT and monoamine oxidase into homovanillic acid. The receptors associated with dopamine are metabotrophic and coupled to G-protein.

33. E COMT

Monoamines are degraded in the synapse as well the presynaptic vesicles. COMT is an enzyme that degrades monoamines such as dopamine, noradrenaline and adrenaline in the synapse. It is encoded by the COMT gene. Dopamine is converted to noradrenaline by dopamine β-hydroxylase. Acetyl-coenzyme A facilitates in production of acetylcholine from choline. Alcohol dehydrogenase and aldehyde dehydrogenase are responsible for the disulfiram reaction.

34. C Aldehyde dehydrogenase

Alcohol is normally metabolised in the liver by the enzyme alcohol dehydrogenase to acetaldehyde. This is further metabolised by the enzyme acetaldehyde dehydrogenase to harmless acetic acid. Disulfiram, Antabuse, inhibits acetaldehyde dehydrogenase with a resultant increase in acetaldehyde. This increase in acetaldehyde is characterised by symptoms such as flushing, palpitations and a throbbing headache, confusion, shortness of breath and collapse. Disulfiram should not be taken within 12 hours of alcohol ingestion.

35. A Basal ganglia

Leigh's disease is a rare and fatal neurodegenerative disease affecting the mitochondria. It is usually seen in children between the age of 3 months and 2 years. On investigations such as MRI and CT, there is evidence of symmetrical necrosis in the brain stem, basal ganglia, medulla oblongata, midbrain and putamen. MR spectroscopy shows elevated choline and lactate. Histologically, Leigh's disease resembles Wernicke's encephalopathy.

36. E Single photon emission computed tomography

This uses manufactured radioactive compounds to study the regional differences in the cerebral blood flow within the brain area. It is a high-resolution imaging technique, which is used to record the pattern of photon emission from the bloodstream. It is based on the level of perfusion in different areas of the brain.

37. D Reduced blood flow in occipital lobe

In dementia with Lewy bodies SPECT will show a reduction in blood flow in the posterior part of the brain, mainly the occipital lobe. The medial temporal lobes are relatively spared. As the illness advances, there can be a global reduction the blood flow. In the early stages of Alzheimer's disease, SPECT will show reduced cerebral blood blow in the parietal and temporal lobes, with relative sparing of the frontal and occipital lobes. In vascular or multi-infarct dementia, SPECT will show a variable and multifocal deficit depending on the site and extent of the infarct or lesion. In depression and Korsakoff's psychosis there is a marked deficit in the frontal area.

38. C Reduced phospholipids in the frontal lobe

In schizophrenia, the following findings are seen consistently on neuroimaging:

CT and MRI:

- Lateral and third ventricle enlargement
- Reduced white and grey matter
- Volume reduction in medial temporal lobes; some volume
- Reduction in prefrontal lobe

MR spectroscopy:

- Reduced concentration of phospholipids and *N*-acetylaspartate in frontal and temporal lobes

Functional imaging:

- Reduced activation of dorsolateral prefrontal cortex 'hypofrontality'
- Striatal hyperdopaminergia.

39. C Protons

Structural MRI constructs images by using the electromagnetic properties of the protons, usually the hydrogen nucleus in water. It has three main types of MRI sequences, namely T1-, T2- and proton-density-weighted images. The most common type of functional MRI (fMRI) involves a blood oxygen level-dependent technique that uses the magnetic properties of deoxygenated and oxygenated haemoglobin. SPECT is an emission rather than a transmission scan. It makes use of γ-rays emitted by an injected radioisotope in the brain and is detected by the γ camera. Positron emission tomography (PET) also makes uses of radioisotopes, but produces images of its distribution in the brain. It is used to measure cerebral blood flow, glucose metabolism, oxygen extraction fraction and blood volume.

40. A Diabetes mellitus

Several antidepressants can cause hyponatraemia, probably via the mechanism of the syndrome of inappropriate secretion of antidiuretic hormone (SIADH). The risk factors for hyponatraemia are old age, female gender, low body weight, low baseline sodium concentration, warm weather and co-administration of drugs such as diuretics, non-steroidal anti-inflammatory drugs, carbamazepine and chemotherapy. Medical comorbidities such as hypothyroidism, diabetes, chronic obstructive pulmonary disease, hypertension, renal failure, head injury and various malignancies are other risk factors for a patient to develop hyponatraemia while on antidepressants.

41. B Aldehyde dehydrogenase 2 deficiency

Alcohol is metabolised by two main enzymes: alcohol dehydrogenase, which converts alcohol to acetaldehyde, and aldehyde dehydrogenase, which converts acetaldehyde to acetate. An aldehyde dehydrogenase type 2 deficiency has been noted in nearly half the Asian population including Chinese and Japanese. Due to deficiency of this enzyme, when alcohol is consumed, there is an accumulation of acetaldehyde in the body. This results in oriental flush syndrome characterised by unpleasant symptoms such as flushing (mainly the face but may involve other parts of the body), tachycardia, diaphoresis, headache, nausea, muscle weakness and sometimes euphoria.

42. C A blood test done 13 hours after the last night dose on day 10 of starting lithium carbonate, while administering the morning dose on time

Blood samples for lithium levels should be taken 10–14 hours post-dose if necessary. It takes 4–5 days for serum lithium levels to reach a steady-state concentration. For trough or pre-dose samples, the blood sample is obtained immediately before the next dose is due. Withholding the next dose for more than 1–2 hours until the sample is taken leads to a misleading result, such as low serum lithium levels.

43. B Discontinuation syndrome

In this patient, given the history, the most likely diagnosis is antidepressant discontinuation syndrome. This is seen with most of the antidepressants, in particular in drugs with a short half-life such as paroxetine and venlafaxine. Abrupt withdrawal of the drug can lead to discontinuation syndrome. Other risk factors for this syndrome include: (1) people taking antidepressants for more than 8 weeks, (2) those patients who had anxiety symptoms at the start of antidepressant therapy, (3) patients who receive other centrally acting medication such as antihypertensives, antipsychotics and antihistamines, (d) past history of discontinuation syndrome, and (e) children and adolescents.

44. A Cross-taper fluoxetine with mirtazapine cautiously

According to the National Institute for Health and Care Excellence (NICE) guidelines, a cautious cross-tapering is indicated for switching of fluoxetine to mirtazapine. The latter should be started at mirtazapine 15 mg and fluoxetine gradually reduced in dose. The speed of cross-tapering should be based on the tolerability of an individual patient.

45. E Olanzapine is the preferred antipsychotic drug

Antipsychotic medication such as olanzapine can be used to treat psychosis and mood disturbance. Lorazepam is preferred over diazepam because of its shorter half-life. Lamotrigine carries a risk of life-threatening rash in the baby and hence is avoided. Lithium is present in a high concentration in the breast milk and not preferred if mother is breastfeeding. Valproate (with adequate contraception and caution against risk of hepatotoxicity in the infant) is preferred over lithium if required. Sertraline is recommended by the NICE guidelines for use during breastfeeding. Fluoxetine and citalopram are present in breast milk in high concentrations and hence not preferred in this case. Paroxetine and sertraline are present in low concentrations in breast milk.

46. A Nicotine acetylcholine receptor antagonism

Memantine is an NMDA receptor antagonist and this action is responsible for its therapeutic effect. It is also an antagonist of $_7$-nicotinic acetylcholine receptor (α_7nAChR). Antagonism at this receptor results in worsening of cognitive function in patients with Alzheimer's dementia. Sudden worsening of cognitive symptoms soon after initiation of memantine has been well documented.

47. C α_2-Adrenoreceptor agonism

Clonidine stimulates the α_2-receptors in the hypothalamus. This leads to the release of growth hormone. This effect is blunted in depression and anxiety. Long-term treatment with antidepressants restores the effect of clonidine on the secretion of growth hormone.

48. E Indirectly stimulating 5-HT$_{2A}$ receptors which results in inhibition of dopamine release

In this scenario the patient has symptoms and signs suggestive of akathisia. Akathisia is mainly caused by D$_2$-receptor antagonism which results in reduced dopamine release. Antipsychotic and antiemetic drugs such as domperidone can cause akathisia by D$_2$-receptor antagonism. Other mechanisms that can result in akathisia are stimulation of 5-HT$_{2A}$-receptors, and antagonism of cholinergic muscarinic receptors and β-adrenoreceptors, all of which result in reduced dopamine release. Selective serotonin receptors are known to cause akathisia by indirectly stimulating 5-HT$_{2A}$-receptors.

49. A Blocking NMDA receptors

Ketamine is an NMDA antagonist. It can produce symptoms similar to those seen in schizophrenia in normal volunteers. This observation is consistent with the NMDA-receptor hypofunction hypothesis of schizophrenia. It may block excitotoxicity, but can also result in worsening of the symptoms; therefore, in research a middle path is being aimed at the treatment targeted at increasing glutamate activity to compensate for NMDA hypofunctioning, but without increasing it so much as to become neurotoxic.

50. E Its main site of action is ventral tegmental area

Acamprosate is a derivative of the amino acid taurine. Its main action is inhibition of the neurotransmission of the excitatory glutamate. It also enhances inhibitory GABA neurotransmission and reduces NMDA activity. Its main site of action is the ventral tegmental area. During alcohol withdrawal, after chronic intake of alcohol, a state of glutamate over-activity (even excitotoxicity) and GABA deficiency sets in. These changes can be mitigated by acamprosate.

51. D 200 mg

Antipsychotic depot injections are indicated for maintenance therapy of psychotic disorders. Zuclopenthixol decanoate may be suitable for aggressive and agitated patients. Table 3.2 indicates an approximate equivalent dose of depot antipsychotic medication. However, dose and frequency will need to be titrated according to the individual patient's response.

Table 3.2 Approximate equivalent doses of depot antipsychotics		
Antipsychotic	Dosage (mg)	Interval (weeks)
Flupenthixol decanoate	40	2
Fluphenazine decanoate	25	2
Haloperidol (as decanoate)	100	4
Pipothiazine palmitate	50	4
Zuclopenthixol decanoate	200	2

52. B Duloxetine

The above-mentioned drug is indicated in the treatment of depression and stress urinary incontinence. The action of duloxetine in the treatment of stress urinary incontinence is associated with reuptake inhibition of serotonin and noradrenaline at the presynaptic neuron in Onuf's nucleus of the sacral spinal cord.

53. D Paroxetine

Of all the selective serotonin reuptake inhibitors (SSRIs), paroxetine is the most potent. Similarly, there is higher chance of discontinuation syndrome with paroxetine rather than other SSRIs.

54. E Tardive dyskinesia

Fly-catching tongue is a sign seen in tardive dyskinesia, which can occur after long-term use of antipsychotic medication. Tardive dyskinesia is a serious, disfiguring and often permanent movement disorder. The dyskinetic movement affects any muscle group but most commonly involves perioral movements and involuntary movement of the tongue. The disorder affects 40–50% of patients treated with long-term use of an antipsychotic. It is not a catatonic phenomenon. Cerebrovascular accidents can give rise to movement disorders. However, in a patient who has schizophrenia and on antipsychotic medication, the first differential would be tardive dyskinesia. Positive symptoms of schizophrenia include thought disorders, delusions and hallucinations.

55. B Lamotrigine levels increase due to inhibition of glucuronidation by sodium valproate

Lamotrigine levels increase due to the inhibition of glucuronidation by sodium valproate. Glucuronidation helps to metabolise lamotrigine to inactive water-soluble compounds, aiding its excretion. This process is inhibited by sodium valproate, resulting in increased lamotrigine plasma levels and possibly toxicity. The combination has been associated, in a number of case reports, with the risk of severe dermatological reactions (including toxic epidermal necrolysis and Stevens–Johnson syndrome), tremors and other adverse effects associated with lamotrigine toxicity (e.g. delirium). In addition, lamotrigine may enhance the metabolism of valproic acid, resulting in small, variable changes in valproate plasma concentrations. It is recommended that an adjustment in dose of either or both drugs is required to minimise or avoid the interaction.

56. C Lithium

Angle-closure glaucoma occurs mainly due to blockade in the drainage of aqueous humour as a result of closure of the iridocorneal angle. Some drugs can precipitate or worsen closed-angle glaucoma mainly due to anticholinergic properties or dilatation of the pupil which can close the iridocorneal angle. All the drugs mentioned in the question except lithium can have this side effect.

57. A Bupropion

This is a noradrenaline and dopamine reuptake inhibitor. Serotoninergic activity and anti-dopaminergic activity are mainly responsible for sexual dysfunction. Therefore, most of the antidepressants can cause sexual side effects because they increase serotoninergic activity. Bupropion increases dopaminergic activity and hence is one of the recommended options to treat SSRI-induced sexual dysfunction. Trazodone has the potential of causing priapism, which is a rare but serious sexual dysfunction.

58. C Mirtazapine

Prolactin release is indirectly modulated by serotonin via stimulation of $5-HT_{1C}$- and $5-HT_2$-receptors. In cases where symptomatic hyperprolactinaemia is confirmed a switch to mirtazapine is recommended. Fluoxetine, paroxetine, venlafaxine and duloxetine have been reported to cause galactorrhoea.

59. B Lamotrigine

The clinical presentation is consistent with a diagnosis of bipolar affective disorder type II. In this disorder, the patient has at least one episode of severe depression and one episode of hypomania. According to the NICE and British Association of Psychopharmacology guidelines, lamotrigine should be considered in bipolar affective disorder type II with predominant depressive episodes. There is good evidence to suggest that it is effective in treatment and prophylaxis of depressive symptoms in bipolar depression. Medications such as lithium, valproate, carbamazepine and olanzapine have modest evidence in prophylaxis of bipolar depression.

60. E Quetiapine

Psychosis in patients with Parkinson's disease is a tricky situation to manage. On the one hand, dopaminergic drugs, used to treat Parkinson's disease, may worsen psychosis whereas, on the other, dopamine antagonists, used to treat psychosis, may worsen its symptoms. Therefore, antipsychotics with the least potential for parkinsonian side effects should be used in such situations. Although clozapine is considered a most effective drug to treat psychosis in Parkinson's disease, quetiapine is preferred as a first line because of better tolerability.

61. C Methadone

In this case scenario, the likely cause of death is QTc prolongation. Both quetiapine and methadone can prolong the QTc interval. Hence, one should be very careful in prescribing a combination of antipsychotics and methadone. There are reports of lofexidine causing QTc prolongation but most of these patients were on a combination of lofexidine and methadone. Aripiprazole has the least effect on the QTc interval. Buprenorphine has fewer effects on QTc prolongation compared with methadone. Naltrexone effects on QTc have not been reported.

62. C It is an aldehyde dehydrogenase inhibitor

Disulfiram (Antabuse) blocks the enzyme aldehyde dehydrogenase. This leads to accumulation of acetaldehyde after consumption of alcohol, causing symptoms such as tachycardia, flushing and hypotension. Disulfiram is used in aversion therapy. Disulfiram also blocks dopamine β-hydroxylase, which helps in reducing crack cocaine use in cocaine-dependent individuals.

63. B Metabotrophic postsynaptic glutamate receptors agonists have shown improvements in symptoms of schizophrenia

The glutamate system is currently being studied to explain the pathophysiology of schizophrenia and discover its treatment. According to this hypothesis, early in the illness, excessive glutamate activity could lead to excitotoxicity and thus interfere with normal neural development. Later on, it may contribute to disease progression in schizophrenia. However, once the schizophrenia has developed, NMDA glutamate receptors are actually hypofunctional. Therefore, both glutamate agonists and antagonists are considered for treatment, depending on the stage of the illness. For the same reason, potent NMDA antagonists might block excitotoxicity, but may worsen symptoms of schizophrenia (e.g. NMDA antagonists such as phencyclidine). Therefore, partial NMDA blockers (amantadine and memantine) could be better options. Metabotrophic presynaptic (not postsynaptic) glutamate receptor-selective agonists, which reduce glutamate release, have shown improvements in symptoms of schizophrenia.

64. C LY404039 can reverse PCP-induced behavioural changes in animals

The glutamate hypothesis of schizophrenia and NMDA receptors is the current focus of research to develop new treatment options for schizophrenia. Agonists at the glycine site of NMDA receptors (e.g. amino acids glycine and D-serine and D-cycloserine, an analogue of D-serine) may boost NMDA-receptor activity just enough to improve symptoms. Glycine transporter-1 (GlyT1) terminates the action of glycine in the synapses. Therefore, their inhibitors increase synaptic availability of glycine and thus enhance NMDA transmission. N-Methyl-glycine, also known as sarcosine, is a naturally occurring GlyT1 inhibitor. This improves negative, affective and cognitive symptoms of schizophrenia. Metabotrophic presynaptic glutamate receptor (mGluRs 2/3) selective agonists (e.g. LY404039) can potentially stop glutamate release and hence have shown improvements in symptoms of schizophrenia. These agents have shown to reverse the behavioural changes induced by the NMDA antagonist PCP in animal experiments. These novel approaches have shown that schizophrenia can potentially be treated without targeting dopamine receptors.

65. C People with the Met genotype of COMT have higher dopamine levels

COMT, which is coded by a gene COMT, has Val158Met as one of the alleles. **Table 3.3** describes the effect of the Met and Val genotype on COMT and dopamine, and its clinical implication.

Table 3.3 Met genotypes of COMT			
Genotype of COMT	Effect on level of COMT activity	Effect on dopamine levels	Clinical implication
Met genotype	Lower COMT activity	Higher	Normal cognitive performance
			Less risk of schizophrenia
			Excessive dopamine release in reaction to stress increases the risk of worry and anxiety disorders
Val genotype	Higher COMT activity	Lower	Reduced cognitive efficiency
			Increased risk of schizophrenia
			Less reactive to stress, less risk of anxiety disorders

66. D Interphase

The cell division cycle of a cell meiotic phase is short-lived and it alternates with a much longer period called interphase. The interphase consists of three phases: A-G one phase, S phase and G2 phase. The cells that are committed to cell division enter the S phase. Mitosis has five stages: interphase, prophase, metaphase, anaphase and telophase. Meiosis in the reproductive cells is where the cell division happens in two stages, resulting in the haploid gamete stage. Except for the interphase, all the stages of mitosis are repeated.

67. C Functional analysis

This is an investigation of gene function by genetic manipulation in animals. It uses techniques such as gene knockout in which one of the organism's genes is made ineffective. The 'knocked-out' organism is then compared with the normal organism to infer important differences. When two or three genes are knocked out, it is called double knockout and triple knockout respectively.

68. C Excises large portions of tRNA during transcription

DNA is transcribed into RNA which is then translated into protein. An RNA-splicing enzyme excises large portions of tRNA while transcribing and modifying of the ends of the RNA molecule (polyadenylation of one end and capping of the other).The final product, which is mRNA, has a central section translated into proteins with non-coding regions in the flanks. So the section of DNA that encodes mRNA, called an exon, is often interrupted by non-translated DNAs called introns.

69. A Chromatin remodelling

A possible mechanism to bring about persistent genetic change in response to environmental stressors is via chromatin remodelling. This is an epigenetic process that modifies DNA. For example, a heritable difference in reaction to stress in rats depends on parenting rather than on DNA. Chromatin remodelling involves either the movement of a nucleosome along the length of the DNA molecule, a process known as 'nucleosome sliding', or chromatin remodellers causing disruption and reorganisation of the nucleosome core, which then makes the DNA available for transcription

70. C Imprinting

Imprinting is another epigenetic system in which a certain gene is active only when it passes to a child via the sperm or ovum. Genomic imprinting is the phenomenon whereby there is a difference of expression of genes depending on whether the chromosomes are from the maternal or the paternal side. DNA methylation represses gene expression. It is reversible and does not affect the DNA sequence itself, but methylation status is maintained when the cells divide, which is referred to as epigenetic modification. DNA methylation is critical for imprinting

71. E Synapsis

Synapsis, also known as syndesis, is basically the pairing of two homologous chromosomes that occurs during meiosis before the non-sister chromatids from opposite chromosomes 'cross-over' (also called 'recombination'), resulting in an exchange of genes that causes a reorganisation and thus increases genetic variability in the next generation. During the first meiotic division in gamete formation, the two coexisting alleles responsible for a specific trait segregate (mendelian law of segregation) or separate, so that each gamete gets only one of the two alleles. These alleles again unite randomly at fertilisation of gametes. The random assortment of maternal and paternal chromosomes in the process of gamete formation leads to 'independent assortment', in other words alleles of different genes assort independently (i.e. randomly) of each other during gamete formation (mendelian law of independent assortment), although sometimes when two genetic loci are too close it results in genetic linkage.

72. E White blood cells

White blood cells are readily accessible and rapidly multiply in a culture. They are therefore the best source for chromosomal analysis. In a culture, they are stimulated by agents such as colchicine. This stops the mitosis in metaphase and cells in metaphase accumulate in the culture. The cells are then fixed and stained. Skin biopsies are for longer-term chromosome culture. Fetal cells from amniocentesis can also be used for culture. Red blood cells do not have chromosomes.

73. C Alterations in the number of sex chromosomes or autosomes

Karyotyping is used to stain and study various chromosomes spread under a microscope. It can detect various chromosomal abnormalities, especially aneuploidies which are basically alterations in the number of sex chromosomes or autosomes. Chromosomal breakage can lead to deletions in which a chromosome may lose a segment, inversion when a segment of chromosome is detached and then reattached in the opposite orientation, and duplication when a segment of a chromosome is included twice over.

74. B Fusion of two chromosomes at their centromere

Rearrangement of parts between non-homologous chromosomes is the process called translocation. Exchange of segments between two different pairs of chromosomes is called reciprocal or non-robertsonian translocation; when two chromosomes fuse at their centromere, it is called robertsonian translocation. The International System for Human Cytogenetic Nomenclature is used to express chromosomal translocations.

75. A Dynamic mutation

Anticipation is a phenomenon whereby the severity of an inherited disease increases and the age of onset decreases in the generations that follow. It occurs due to an unstable DNA sequence in dynamic mutation; trinucleotide repeat disorders are seen in this type of mutation. Examples of trinucleotide repeat disorder are fragile X syndrome, Friedreich's ataxia, myotonic dystrophy, Huntington's disease and, spinobulbar muscular atrophy.

Anticipation is seen well in Prader–Willi syndrome where seven genes on paternal chromosome 15 (q11-13) are deleted or unexpressed and also in Angelman's syndrome where it is the maternal chromosome that is involved, i.e. seven genes on maternal chromosome 15 (q11-13) are deleted or unexpressed.

76. A DNA methylation

This represses gene expression. Methylation of DNA is reversible and it does not affect the DNA sequence itself although the methylation status is maintained when the cells divide, which is referred to as epigenetic modification. DNA methylation is critical for imprinting. Transcription factors control gene expression. Pleiotropy is mutation in transcription factors. A reverse transcriptase (or RNA-dependent DNA polymerase) is a DNA polymerase enzyme that basically transcribes a single-stranded RNA into a single stranded DNA.

77. E No case occurring in previous generation, but the disease may manifest in children of next generation

In autosomal recessive disorders, if both the parents carry one copy of the mutant gene, then they won't manifest the disorder. However, one in four of their children will be affected. This phenomenon in which the disorder skips a generation is called horizontal transmission.

78. D Single nucleotide polymorphism

Genetic markers are described as variation in the DNA length or sequence that can be observed. They are very helpful in gene mapping. First of these to be discovered was restriction fragment length polymorphism (RFLP) which has largely been replaced by single nucleotide polymorphism. Informative combination of genetic markers is known as a haplotype. The methods for mapping are association and linkage.

79. C Environmental factors by biological mechanism

The above mentioned is an example of gene regulation by environmental factors using a biological mechanism. These effects may persist over two generations and appear possibly reversible. Activity and expression of a gene are regulated by environmental factors such as psychosocial stressors, inherited DNA or RNA, endogenous factors such as hormones and a non-inherited mechanism known as epigenetics. Epigenetics is the study of molecular mechanisms in gene expression or cellular phenotype due to mechanisms other than changes in the underlying DNA/RNA sequence, e.g. DNA methylation or histone acetylation.

80. E Genetic linkage

Genetic linkage is investigating the co-segregation of the disease and a set of genetic markers while studying disease in families. The aim of linkage analysis is to determine the location of the gene(s) on a chromosome for a trait of interest, e.g. a common disease. The purpose of genetic algorithms is to generate solutions to problems by giving due consideration to the processes as they may occur in nature, i.e. natural evolution, inheritance, mutation, selection, recombination and mutation. DNA or RNA has some sequence of nucleotides that in turn controls the amino acid sequence in the protein to be generated by that particular sequence of nucleotides. To study sequence of codons (single unit of three adjacent nucleotides in DNA or RNA) is called genetic coding.

81. E It is zero when the two loci are very close together

A recombinant fraction is the number of recombinants divided by the total number of offspring and is the most important parameter. In linkage studies genetic distance is expressed in centimorgans (cM). The recombinant fraction is zero when the two loci are very close together. If two loci are widely apart, independent assortment occurs and recombination fraction = 1/2. A recombination fraction is just a numerical value and does not have any units. A recombination occurs more in female than in male meiosis. The recombination fraction at any locus is the proportion of meiotic products that are non-parental recombinant.

82. E 3

In linkage analysis, the logarithm of the odd (LOD) is the log of the odds that the recombinant fraction (RF) has a certain value. A LOD score of 3 or more indicates that linkage has been detected. A LOD of −2 or less excludes linkage at that particular value of RF and that a LOD of 3+ indicates 1000: 1 odds that the linkage observed is not by chance.

83. A Genetic variation in a population will remain constant from one generation to the next in the absence of disturbing factors

The Hardy–Weinberg equilibrium states that allele and genotype variation in a population remains constant between generations if there are no factors that may cause disturbance. Factors that may introduce disturbance in the Hardy–Weinberg equilibrium include selection, mutations, gene flow, gene drift and mating. Mutation can introduce disturbance by adding new alleles to the population which may be passed to another generation.

84. B Gene flow

Gene flow (also known as gene migration) is when there is mating between diverse populations, probably due to migration; a certain disturbance is introduced that causes a change in the combination and frequency of alleles. Genetic drift is a change that occurs in the number of alleles (gene variant) due to random sampling in a population over time. Random mating is when allele combinations happen by chance without disturbance from social, environmental or other factors. Genetic recombination and independent assortment are concepts described in relation to cell division.

85. D Nicotinic receptor gene

There is on-going research to link the endophenotype to genes. P50 suppression studies have shown a specific linkage of P50 suppression with a genetic marker at the locus of the α_7-subunit of the nicotinic receptor gene.

86. D 50%

Schizophrenia is a highly heritable condition. The chances of an offspring developing schizophrenia when the parents have schizophrenia are up to 50%.

87. B More than four-fifths of the variance in causes of schizophrenia are genetically determined

For genetic studies in schizophrenia, sampling is done in two stages. In stage 1, a random sample of the people with schizophrenia is obtained; they are called index cases or 'probands'. In stage 2, relatives of the probands are assessed for the presence (if present, called 'secondary cases') or absence of schizophrenia. Monozygotic (MZ) twins are developed from the same fertilised ovum and are therefore genetically identical; dizygotic (DZ) twins are developed from two separate fertilised ova, thus sharing 50% of their genetic material. The risk of a disease in a relative of a proband is called 'morbid risk' or 'recurrence risk'. As the criteria are slightly different the pooled MZ and DZ rates were 50% and 4% using the DSM-IV and 42% and 4% respectively when using the ICD-10 criteria. More than four-fifths of the variance in cause of schizophrenia is genetically determined. Probandwise the concordance rate is defined as the percentage of probands who have an affected co-twin. MZ probandwise concordance rate is around 46% and DZ probandwise concordance rate is around 4%.

88. A Among female siblings of patients with established anorexia nervosa (AN), 5–10% of them have the condition compared with 0.5–1.0% found in the general population of the same age

Concordance rate for AN in MZ twins is 55% and in DZ twins 5%. Siblings of patients with AN have increased chances of bulimia nervosa and eating disorder not otherwise specified. This increase in risk might be due to family environment or genetic influence. Some association studies done in AN have indicated a polymorphism in the promoter region of the 5-HT$_{2A}$-receptor. The concordance rate in DZ twins is only 5%. Inherited liability to AN might involve relevant personality traits such as perfectionism and obsessionality. There is an association between eating disorders and mood disorders. Among female siblings of patients with established AN, 5–10% have the condition compared with 0.5–1.0% in the general population of the same age. Weak genetic linkage is on a site on chromosome 1p. Epigenetic mechanisms may contribute to the alterations of atrial natriuretic peptide homeostasis in females with eating disorders. The *BDNF* gene on chromosome 11 may show polymorphism contributing to susceptibility to AN.

89. A In unipolar depression, the concordance rate is 46% in MZ and 20% in DZ twins

The concordance rate of both unipolar and bipolar depression in DZ twins is 20%. The concordance rate of unipolar depression in MZ twins is around 46%. Bipolar depression has more heritability than unipolar depression. Genetic factors play a more important role in females and thus there is a high female preponderance in depression. The genetic contribution is via polygenic inheritance, i.e. several genes of small effect acting together. Linkages involving chromosomes 13q and 22q are seen in bipolar affective disorder. A particular serotonin transporter allele has been found in association studies which increases the vulnerability of the patient for a major depressive episode when encountered with a stressful life event. Overall the genetic influence in bipolar is higher than in unipolar disorder. Relatives of patients with unipolar depression do not have increased risk of bipolar or schizoaffective disorder. The concordance rate for mood disorders in MZ twins is between 60 and 70%, and for DZ twins the rate is about 20%.

90. D Urban areas

According to Finnish twin studies, the drinking rate was similar in adolescents living in rural and urban areas. However, in urban areas, gene-related factors had a greater influence on drinking rate in adolescents whereas in a rural setting it was found to be environment and related factors. Furthermore, the influence of genetic factors was observed to be five times higher where there was higher migration, younger population, and greater alcohol availability and sale.

91. E Stressful life events that involve a threat lead to GAD

Roy et al, in their study on a clinical sample of twins, concluded that major depression was associated with stressful life events that involved loss, whereas threat or danger was a significant life event leading to generalised anxiety disorder. This sample included both males and females.

92. A Gene–environment correlation

In gene–environment interaction, environmental factors are difficult to define and understudied. Some putative environmental factors may not be truly environmental. In such situations an individual's genotype influences his exposure to the environment. This is called gene–environment correlation.

93. D Susceptibility gene

In disorders where the cause is multifactorial, a single gene is neither necessary nor sufficient for the development of disorders. For example, ε4 is a susceptibility gene for the development of Alzheimer's disease. However, it is neither sufficient nor necessary for the development of Alzheimer's dementia. Even though it can be seen to increase the risk, it is called a 'susceptibility gene'.

94. E Presence of one ε4 allele and past history of head injury

Studies on Alzheimer's disease (AD) have shown the following results. A positive family history of AD alone does not increase the risk of developing it. Again a past history of head injury alone does not increase the risk of developing AD in the absence of the ε4 allele. ε2/ε3 does not increase the susceptibility for developing AD. A two fold risk of developing AD is seen with the presence of the ε4 allele. However, some studies have shown that this effect decreases after the age of 70 years. There is a 10-fold increase in the risk of developing AD in people who are positive for the ε4 allele and have a past history of head injury.

95. C 7%

Population-based studies estimate a prevalence of 7% of autism in learning disability. For the other illnesses the prevalence is as follows:

Schizophrenia: 3%

Bipolar affective disorder: 1.5%

Depression: 4%

Dementia at age 65 years or above: 20%.

96. C 3%

The prevalence of schizophrenia in learning disability is 3%. This may be an understatement because the general population prevalence is 1%.

97. D 0.7

Coid et al (2003) describe the prevalence of personality disorders in the community. Some of the prevalence rates are as follows:

Schizotypal: 0.1–5.6%

Schizoid: 0.4–1.7%

Antisocial: 0.6–3.0%

Borderline: 0.7–2.0%

Narcissistic: 0.4–0.8%

Histrionic: 2.1%

Paranoid: 0.7–2.4%

Avoidant: 0.8–5.0%

Dependent: 1.0–1.7%

Compulsive: 1.7–2.2%

All personality disorders: 4.4–13 %. The prevalence of borderline personality disorder among psychiatric inpatients is 15%.

98. C 3–6%

Developmental dyslexia is a specific impairment in learning to read and is also called specific reading disorder. It affects about 3–6% of school age children in English-speaking countries.

99. E 53%

Young et al (2006) concluded that identification as belonging to Goth subculture was strongly associated with a lifetime prevalence rate of 53% for self-harm and 47% for attempted suicide. There was a dose–response relation. Even after adjusting for confounders and comparing with other subcultures this was significant.

100. A 4–5%

The life-time prevalence of suicide in schizophrenia is about 10 times higher than in the general population. In particular, higher suicide risk is found in young adults. Initial studies suggested that the life-time risk of 13%. However, more recent studies suggest a life-time risk of 4–5% taking into account the variability in the rate in different age groups. Over time a reduction in suicide rate is found similar to the general population.

101. C 0.3%

The estimated prevalence rate of anorexia nervosa is 0.3% and for bulimia nervosa it is 1%. Males have approximately a tenth the incidence rates.

102. C 13 per 100,000 persons per year

The registered incidence rate for bulimia nervosa is 13 per 100,000 persons per year and for anorexia nervosa is 8 per 100,000 persons per year. A third of people diagnosed with anorexia and 6% of those diagnosed with bulimia nervosa are treated in mental health care.

103. C 12%

The EURODEP study gathered data from nine European centres. It concluded that the prevalence of depression in old people aged > 65 years is 12.3% for both men and women combined. For women, it is 14.1% and for men 8.6%.

104. D 1 in 20

Coid et al (2006) found that 1 in 20 community residents in Britain has a personality disorder. Certain demographic groups have a higher prevalence of personality disorder.

105. C It is more prevalent in men than in women

Vascular dementia is the second commonest cause of dementia after Alzheimer's dementia. It accounts for 10–50% case of dementia depending on factors such as geographical location, clinical methods used for diagnosis and the patient population. The incidence varies from 1.2% to 4.2% in those aged > 65 years and 6–12 cases per1000 aged > 70 years per year. Prevalence and incidence increase with age, men having a higher incidence than women. The prevalence had been higher in recent series comprising older individuals. Stroke and cerebrovascular disorders cause higher cognitive impairment and dementia. Vascular factors may in fact be the leading cause of 'cognitive impairment' rather than Alzheimer's disease, if dementia is not considered as a cause of cognitive impairment.

106. B Association of schizophrenia is seen with maternal age in patients with no family history of schizophrenia

As paternal age is an independent risk factor for schizophrenia, even after controlling for family history, it indicates that the reason might be a cumulative effect of new mutations in sperm due to ageing.

107. B Many studies have shown that schizoaffective disorder has a better course than schizophrenia but poorer than affective disorders

Schizoaffective disorders with poor outcomes are due to a higher number of cycles, poor interepisode recovery, and persisting psychosis in the absence of affective features, and the presence of mixed state, chronicity, poor premorbid level of social adjustment and more schizophrenia-like symptoms.

108. E Sri Lanka

The suicide rate in Sri Lanka, Lithuania, China, Japan and Belarus was 16.8, 16.1, 14.8, 14.1 and 9.5 respectively.

109. B 15 to 44-year-old males

In UK from 2000 to 2009 the suicide rate was found to be highest among 15 to 44-year-old males.

110. E 75+ years

In people aged > 75 years, the rate of suicide was 50.0 for males and 15.8 for females in the global WHO distribution for age and gender.

111. C 4

Infant mortality rate is the number of deaths of children under the age of 1 year per 1000 live births. In this case, it will be 4 per 1000 live births.

112. C Morgan–Russell assessment schedule

This is often used in long-term outcome studies of eating disorders.

Bech–Rafaelsen rating scale: there is a scale for mania and another for melancholia. The scale for mania is used to assess the presence and severity of clinical features of mania/hypomania and the effectiveness of therapeutic interventions for bipolar disorders. The scale for melancholia is useful when severe depression is also measured.

Conners' rating scale: this is used for assessment of attention deficit hyperactivity disorder (ADHD) in children and adolescents. There is a Conners' rating scale for adult ADHD as well.

Vanderbilt assessment scale: used for ADHD assessment in children.

Wender–Utah rating scale is used for assessment of adult ADHD. It focuses on childhood and current symptoms.

113. D 5

The odds ratio is a ratio of the odds occurring in the exposed (experimental) group compared with the odds of the same event occurring in the placebo (control) group.

Odds ratio = odds of events occurring in exposed or odds of events occurring in non-exposed

Odds ratio = 1: suggests that exposure has no effect when compared with non-exposed group

Odds ratio > 1: suggests exposure increased the outcome

Odds ratio > 1 suggests exposure reduced the outcome compared with non-exposed group.

114. A Diagnostic interview schedule

This was first used in a US epidemiological catchment area study. It is a highly structured interview delivered by trained non-clinicians. The other rating scale that is delivered by trained non-clinicians is the composite international diagnostic interview. The other rating scales mentioned in the option are delivered by clinicians.

115. E Prospective

Case registry is a prospective, cumulative collection of databases at a population level. It includes details of demography and limited clinical data, e.g. diagnosis. It is linked to other registers such as birth registries that can give lot more information. It is geographically defined and population based.

116. A Composite international diagnostic interview

This was used in a national comorbidity survey that was the first large-scale survey of mental health in the USA from 1990 to 1992. The composite international diagnostic interview (CIDI) was designed to be used by trained non-clinicians. It can be used as computerised assessments and it gives both ICD-10 and DSM diagnoses. It has questions from both the diagnostic interview schedule (DIS) and present state examination.

DIS was used in the epidemiological catchment area study.

117. A It can be graded into cognitive and somatic subscales

Beck's depression inventory (recent version BDI 2 in 1996) measures the severity of depression rather than its nature. The symptoms mentioned by 21 questions in the BDI can be subdivided into somatic and psychological or cognitive symptoms. It is self-rated and correlates well with the HAM-D score.

118. A [35/50] × 100

Sensitivity = [True positive/(True positive + False negative)] × 100.

119. C [9940/9950] × 100

Specifity = [True negative/(True negative + False positive)] × 100.

120. E 50/10000

The prevalence is calculated by dividing the number of infected patients by the total number of patients.

121. B (35/45) × 100

Positive predictive value = True positive/(True positive + False positive).

122. C (9940/9950) × 100

Negative predictive value = True negative/(True negative + False negative).

123. C Reward dependence

The psychobiological model of personality by Cloninger includes four dimensions of temperament and three components of character which are shaped by the environment. The temperamental dimensions include novelty seeking, harm avoidance, reward dependence and persistence. The character dimensions are self-directedness, coperativeness and self-transcendence.

124. C Therapeutic community approach is helpful in reducing reoffending after release in offenders with drug and alcohol misuse

The therapeutic community approach, when offered in prison, has been observed to result in a reduction in the recidivism rate after release among offenders who have substance and alcohol misuse. In antisocial personality disorder, comorbidities such as anxiety and axis I disorder are common. Infants who are at risk of developing conduct disorder, when offered interventions that focus on developing parent–child attachment, are found to benefit. There is good evidence for cognitive, behavioural, multi-systemic and functional family therapy in reducing re-offending rate in adolescent with conduct disorder.

125. A Manually assisted cognitive therapy is a type of brief psychological intervention

Brief psychological therapies are defined as low-intensity interventions delivered for less than 6 months. Manually assisted cognitive therapy (MACT) is a type of brief psychological intervention. The evidence base for brief psychological therapies is limited to MACT with only two randomized controlled trials known so far. Cost-effectiveness varies between studies identified when compared with usual treatment.

126. B Non-RCT evidence suggests that individual psychological therapies are well accepted by patients and show positive outcomes

There is limited randomized controlled trial (RCT) evidence for individual psychological interventions. There is weak RCT evidence for critically appraised topics (in young people) and for systems training for emotional predictability and problem solving (STEPPS) in improving general functioning and reducing self-harm. Non-RCT evidence shows positive outcomes and this it is well accepted by patients. CBT, schema-focused psychotherapy and individual psychotherapy have not shown much benefit.

127. B Dialectical strategies encompass aspects of both acceptance and change

The CBT was developed by Linehan for women who self-harm. It has four stages. Weekly individual therapy and a weekly psychoeducational and skills training group are offered concurrently for a contracted period (usually 1 year). Dialectical strategies that encompass aspects of both acceptance and change are an integral feature of the treatment. The therapist is also available to patients out of hours on the phone for 'coaching'.

128. B Medication is prohibited for personality disorders in some therapeutic communities

The ultimate aim of therapeutic community treatment is to rehabilitate individuals. Usually these are weekly residential full-time day units. Most operate a rolling programme of 1–2 years' duration. Medication is prohibited in some communities. Behavioural interventions such as agreeing contracts and consequences for certain behaviours are often included as part of community meetings.

129. D It was devised by Bateman and Fonagy in 2004

Bateman and Fonagy developed metallisation-based therapy (MBT) for patients with borderline personality disorder. MBT is based on psychoanalytic psychotherapy and is effective in reducing self-harm and suicidal behaviour, anger, aggression and depression. When offered with partial hospitalisation, it is delivered for a maximum of 18 months and involves weekly individual analytic therapy and community meetings. A randomised controlled trial comparing 18-month MBT in an outpatient clinic with a standard outpatient clinic was effective in reducing self-harm, suicidal behaviour, need for hospitalisation and other outcomes.

130. B Authoritative

Three main parenting styles are described.

In the authoritative style, the child is encouraged to explore and become independent while consistent parenting and boundaries are set in place.

The authoritarian style is where the parents do not negotiate and are strict. The boundaries set are clear and rigid. The children tend to have a low self-esteem and can be socially withdrawn.

The authoritative style is where the parents discuss and explain to the child so that there are firm rules with shared decision-making. The children are usually sociable and popular and have a positive self-esteem.

The permissive style is where there are few limits set by the parents with no clear guidelines, and the children usually have poor impulse control and display aggression.

131. E To resolve the complex, the boy represses his desires for his mother and his hostile feelings for his father

According to Sigmund Freud, the Oedipus complex starts in the phallic stage which lasts from 3 years to 6 years. The boy takes his mother as the first love object and doesn't wish to share her with the father. He becomes jealous of the father and develops hostile feeling towards him.

He eventually becomes scared that the father may punish him by castrating him. To resolve the difficulty, he represses his desires for the mother and his hostile feelings towards him. He then identifies with the father (aggressor) which helps him develop his super-ego and the male sex role. A similar complex in girls is known as the electra complex wherein she experiences penis envy and turns to her father as the first love object.

132. B Ego

According to Freud the structural model of the mind consists of three areas:

1. Id: instinctual drives and operates under primary processes
2. Ego: logical and abstract thinking with verbal expression
3. Super-ego: it is the conscience and moral values and ideas are held with secondary processes.

133. A Ego

The ego extends through all three topographical domains of the preconscious, conscious and unconscious systems.

134. D Paranoid schizoid position

Klein described the paranoid schizoid position and the depressive position.

- Paranoid schizoid position: it is associated with 'persecutory anxiety' where all aspects of the infant and mother are split into good and bad in the mother.
- Depressive position: here there is mixed ambivalent feelings held about the mother.

135. E Transitional object

Winnicott added to the school of thought of the object relations theory. He proposed the theory of multiple self-organisations (false and true self) which develops in a holding environment that is provided by a good-enough mother. A good-enough mother refers to the idea that the mother does not need to be perfect. The transitional object is a buffer (e.g. blanket or teddy bear) that can be real or fantasy, which helped the infant negotiate separation from the mother to become more independent.

136. D Melanie Klein

Klein proposed theories after observing infants' development and play, and described the stages of the paranoid schizoid position and the depressive position.

Skinner is known for his work with operant conditioning. Rogers was known for proposing the person-centred theory of personality. Jung proposed the concepts of archetypes and the collective unconscious. Sigmund Freud proposed the topographical and structural models of the mind.

137. E Weaning

According to Melanie Klein, during human development, the developmental stage of weaning is symbolically representative of castration to the infant.

138. C Interview measures may be better than self-report measures

Both self-reports and interviews can be used to assess adult attachment styles. Although the self-report method is easy to administer and analyse, and readily available it has theoretical limitations. Training is required to administer the interview method for assessment of adult attachment styles and is better than the self-report method. The semi-structured adult attachment interview was designed by George, Kaplan and Main.

139. C Structure resides in the investigator's conceptualisation of the phenomenon being studied

The investigator-based diagnostic interview usually requires training and resources, and takes time to administer as well as analyse. The structure resides in the investigator's conceptualisation of the phenomenon and probing for descriptions of behaviours. These are usually semi-structured interviews. The behaviours are rated by the investigator who makes the decision whether or not the phenomenon is present. It can be hard to get inter-rater reliability and it is more open to investigator bias.

140. B Lay people can deliver these interviews

These can be delivered by lay members, requires fewer resources and little/no training, and is less time-consuming to deliver. The structure of these interviews resides in the questions being asked in exactly the same way. These interviews are used in epidemiological studies.

141. C Labels can be helpful

In child psychiatry, the ICD-10 does not allow for comorbidity in contrast to the DSM-IV. It is not clear which is preferable. Children who meet the diagnostic criteria may not actually have the problem and many children who have severe impairment may not actually meet the criteria for diagnosis. Labelling can lead to stigma but can be helpful for psychoeducation and increase understanding. There can be an overlap between differential diagnoses.

142. A It can be improved by teaching skills to the parent

The relationship between a parent and a child can be improved by teaching skills to the parent. The relationship is based on principles of operant conditioning and attachment theory. Attachment relationships usually form first to the primary caregiver and then the child goes onto form other attachment relations. The parent–child relationship is regulated by multiple mechanisms. It may or may not be affected by parental mental illness.

143. A It is based on practical considerations

Assessment usually focuses on the entire family relations as well as individuals. The parent, child or both may be present at the interview. The assessment takes into account practical considerations where a child psychiatrist assessing a child should theoretically refer the mother to a general psychiatrist. Maternal psychiatric disorders can cause serious disturbance in a child and be viewed with a lower priority by general psychiatrists. It may be in the child's interest for the child psychiatrist to consider treatment of both the mother and the child.

144. A Distress tolerance

The DBT proposed by Marsha Linehan is based on 'dialectic' which involves changing what needs to be changed while accepting a valid response to a particular situation or circumstance. Elements of therapy involve:

1. Capability enhancement: emotional regulation, distress tolerance and improving interpersonal skills.
2. Motivational enhancement: application of skills developed to life problems.

There are links to CBT methods and Zen Buddhism.

145. B Contemplation

Motivational interviewing, also known as the transtheoretical model, is a patient directive approach which helps to achieve behaviour change. Motivational interviewing has many applications in psychiatry, particularly where there is resistance to change. There are five stages of change in the transtheoretical model developed by Prochaska aned DiClemente. The first stage is precontemplation where an individual is not ready to think about change seriously. In the second stage, contemplation, the individual is ready to think about change. The third stage is determination when an individual starts preparing plans for change. In the fourth stage, action plans are implemented and finally, in the maintenance stage, the individual ensures that the change in behaviour becomes habitual.

Table 3.4 Stages of change	
Precontemplation	Individual is not ready to think about change seriously
Contemplation	Individual is ready to think about change
Determination	Individual is preparing to make plans for change
Action	Individual is implementing change
Maintenance	Individual ensures that the change in behaviour becomes habitual

146. B Selective abstraction

Selective abstraction is an example of cognitive distortion. Some other examples of cognitive distortion are all-or-none thinking, overgeneralisation, magnification, minimisation and jumping to conclusions, to name a few. Metaphor is a term used in cognitive linguistics and metaphor therapy. Splitting is a defence mechanism usually seen in patients with borderline personality disorder. Triangulation has several definitions; however, in psychology it is related to an idea in dysfunctional family dynamics and is described in Bowen's theory. Trap, dilemma and snags are terms used in cognitive–analytical therapy.

147. C Childhood asthma

There is some evidence that systemic therapy can be provided as an adjunct to medication in treatment of childhood asthma. This is of particular benefit when childhood asthma is associated with poor control and/or emotional disturbance. Systemic therapy is also a useful intervention in managing enuresis, oppositional behaviour, and affective, psychotic and eating disorders.

148. D Regression

Table 3.5 The classification of defence mechanisms			
Narcissistic	**Immature**	**Neurotic**	**Mature**
Denial	Acting out	Controlling	Altruism
Distortion	Blocking	Displacement	Anticipation
Projection	Hypochondriasis	Externalisation	Asceticism
	Introjection	Inhibition	Humour
	Passive–aggressive behaviour	Intellectualisation	Sublimation
	Regression	Isolation	Suppression
	Schizoid fantasy	Rationalisation	
	Somatisation	Dissociation	
		Reaction formation	
		Repression	
		Sexualisation	

149. D Rationalisation

The process occurring in the defence mechanisms is listed below:

- Acting out: here the individual behaves in a way to enact the difficult emotions rather than process them internally.
- Altruism: this is a way of avoiding dealing with one's difficult emotions by selflessly doing for others.
- Dissociation: here the patient will separate him- or herself from reality, having no contact with painful experiences.
- Rationalisation: a person will justify his or her thoughts and feelings and experiences using what appear to the individual to be a logical explanation, although this in fact is unrelated.
- Repression: here the individual unconsciously puts difficult experiences out of the mind and therefore does not have to deal with them.

150. E Phobias are maintained by operant conditioning

Classic conditioning is basic form of conditioning also known as pavlovian conditioning. Edward Thorndike suggested the law of effect, which is based around positive and negative reinforcements. Observational (vicarious) learning can also lead to establishment of conditional responses, both classic and operant. Phobias may develop by classic conditioning, but it is hypothesised that phobias, once established, are maintained by operant conditioning.

151. A Cognitive–behaviour therapy

Psychological interventions such as CBT, behavioural therapies or social network- and environment-based therapies should be offered to people with harmful drinking and mild alcohol dependence. Such therapies should also be offered after successful withdrawal from moderate-to-severe alcohol dependence. Family therapy should be considered in children and adolescents with alcohol misuse.

152. D Multidimensional family therapy should consist of 12–15 sessions

Psychological treatment in children and young people who abuse alcohol can be provided by multidimensional family therapy or brief strategic family therapy. Multidimensional therapy is provided over 12 weeks and includes 12–15 structured sessions aimed at reducing substance misuse, education, improving behaviour, parenting skills and wellbeing. Brief strategic family therapy is provided over 12 weeks with fortnightly meetings.

153. D McCord and McCord

McCord and McCord (1964) described 'guiltlessness' and 'lovelessness' being the essence of psychopathy. Parental neglect and rejection were aetiologically linked to development of these core characteristics of psychopathy. McCord and McCord also described psychopaths as cold, violent and predatory.

154. A Boys show more deprivation features than girls

Table 3.6 Early life experiences in children	
Rutter studied early life adversity in children, in particular privation and deprivation	
Deprivation	Privation
Attachment here is formed and lost	No attachment is formed
Seen after harsh and aggressive parenting and physical abuse	Rare occurrence
Features seen more common in boys than girls	Can lead to affectionless psychopathy

Question: MCQs

For each question, select one answer option.

NEUROSCIENCES: NEUROANATOMY

1. In which part of the brain are mammillary bodies located?

   A   Caudate
   B   Hypothalamus
   C   Pigmented part of substantia nigra
   D   Putamen
   E   Ventral striatum

2. Where do the anterior thalamic nuclei receive their afferents from?

   A   Cerebellum
   B   Globus pallidus
   C   Inferior colliculus
   D   Mammillary body
   E   Superior colliculus

3. A 39-year-old man has partial optic nerve damage. Which visual field defect is most likely to occur?

   A   Bilateral central scotomas
   B   Bitemporal hemianopia
   C   Homonymous hemianopia
   D   Homonymous upper quadrantanopia
   E   Ipsilateral scotoma

4. A 45-year-old woman developed homonymous upper quadrantanopia. Where is the lesion most likely to be located in the visual pathway?

   A   Bilateral macular cortex
   B   Meyer's loop
   C   Optic chiasma
   D   Optic radiation
   E   Visual cortex

5. In which part of the frontal lobe is Broca's area situated?

   A   Dorsolateral prefrontal cortex
   B   Frontal operculum
   C   Inferior mesial region
   D   Superior mesial region
   E   Superior temporal gurus

6.   Where does the hypothalamus originate from?

   A   Corpus striatum
   B   Diencephalon
   C   Midbrain
   D   Pons
   E   Telencephalon

7.   Which of the following consists of the basal forebrain?

   A   Dorsolateral prefrontal cortex
   B   Frontal operculum
   C   Inferior mesial region
   D   Superior mesial region
   E   Superior temporal gurus

8.   Which of the following cranial nerve fibres terminates in the anterior and posterior cochlear nuclei?

   A   Accessory nerve
   B   Glossopharyngeal nerve
   C   Hypoglossal nerve
   D   Vagus nerve
   E   Vestibulocochlear nerve

9.   Which of the following is a part of the cortical area of the limbic lobe?

   A   Amygdaloid nucleus
   B   Cingulate gyrus
   C   Hypothalamus
   D   Olfactory bulb
   E   Septal nucleus

NEUROSCIENCES: NEUROPATHOLOGY

10.   A 54-year-old woman presents with multiple intracranial and spinal tumours, mainly schwannomas and neurofibromas. What is the most likely diagnosis?

   A   Bilateral acoustic neurofibromatosis
   B   Sturge–Weber syndrome
   C   Tuberous sclerosis
   D   Von Hippel–Lindau disease
   E   Von Recklinghausen's neurofibromatosis

11.   Which of the following is a characteristic feature of frontotemporal dementia?

   A   Global brain atrophy
   B   Knife blade gyri
   C   Pick's bodies
   D   Sulcal widening
   E   Ventricular enlargement

12.   Which of the following are the characteristic macroscopic changes seen in multi-infarct dementia?

   A   Arteriosclerotic changes in major arteries
   B   Global brain atrophy
   C   Knife blade gyri

D   Sulcal widening
E   Ventricular enlargement

13. Which of the following are the characteristic histopathological changes seen in Lewy body dementia?

A   Arteriosclerotic changes in major arteries
B   Changes including infarction and ischaemia
C   Local or general brain atrophy
D   Neuritic plaques
E   Sulcal widening

14. Which of the following tumours are embryonal in origin?

A   Gliomas
B   Haemangioblastomas
C   Medulloblastomas
D   Meningeal tumours
E   Pituitary adenomas

15. Which of the following is a characteristic feature of Prion disease?

A   Amyloid plaques containing β-amyloid protein
B   Amyloid plaques containing prion protein (PrP)
C   Amyloid plaques containing PrP and β-amyloid protein
D   Gliosis which is rarely seen in prion disease
E   Neuronal amount usually maintained

NEUROSCIENCES: NEUROPHYSIOLOGY

16. Secretion of which of the following hormones is inhibited by dopamine?

A   Adrenocorticotrophic hormone
B   Follicle-stimulating hormone
C   Growth hormone
D   Prolactin
E   Thyroid-stimulating hormone

17. Which of the following is an inhibitory hypothalamic hormone?

A   Arginine vasopressin
B   Corticotrophin-releasing hormone
C   Gonadotrophin-releasing hormone
D   Growth hormone-releasing hormone
E   Somatostatin

18. Which of the following receptors is linked with a moderate (10–100 m/s) second messenger?

A μ
B δ
C κ
D α_1
E   Cholecystokinin A

19. Which group of nerve fibres innervates tendon organs?

    A   Ia
    B   Ib
    C   II
    D   III
    E   IV

20. Which of the following statements about neuronal action potential is correct?

    A   Action potential is conducted along axons with decrement
    B   Closing of potassium channels is associated with repolarisation
    C   Conduction is independent of the resistance and conductance of the membrane
    D   During the action potential the neuronal membrane can be stimulated
    E   Influx of sodium into the cell leads to depolarisation

NEUROSCIENCES: NEUROENDOCRINOLOGY

21. Which of the neurohormones stimulates growth hormone release?

    A   Arginine vasopressin
    B   β-Endorphin
    C   Cortisol
    D   Oxytocin
    E   Somatostatin

NEUROSCIENCES: NEUROCHEMISTRY

22. Which of the following is the precursor in the synthesis of acetylcholine?

    A   Choline
    B   Dopamine β-hydroxylase
    C   Histidine
    D   L-Tryptophan
    E   L-Tyrosine

23. Which of the following best describes γ-aminobutyric acid A receptors?

    A   G-protein coupled
    B   Ligand-gated ion channel
    C   Metabotrophic
    D   Steroid and thyroid hormone like
    E   Tyrosine kinase linked

24. What changes have been reported on pre- and postmortem studies of patients with depression?

    A   Decreased 5-hydroxytryptamine 2-receptors in limbic areas
    B   Decreased muscarinic receptors in limbic area
    C   Increased β-adrenoreceptors in cortical areas
    D   Increased 5-HIAA in cerebrospinal fluid
    E   Increased nicotinic receptors in cortical area

25. Which of the following is a precursor in the synthesis of dopamine?

   A   Adrenaline
   B   Choline esterase
   C   L-Tyrosine
   D   Noradrenaline
   E   Tryptophan

26. Which of the following neurotransmitters was discovered first?

   A   Biogenic amines
   B   γ-Aminobutyric acid
   C   Glycine
   D   Neurotensin
   E   Peptides

NEUROSCIENCES: NEUROIMAGING

27. A 70-year-old man was diagnosed with vascular dementia. Which of the following diagnostic systems does not require neuroimaging for vascular dementia?

   A   California criteria
   B   *Diagnostic and Statistical Manual of Mental Disorders*, 4th edn (DSM-IV)
   C   Hachinski's scale
   D   The ICD-10 (*International Classification of Diseases*, 10th revision)
   E   NINDS/AIREN (National Institute of Neurological Disorders and Stroke and Association Internationale pour la Recherché et l'Enseignement en Neurosciences) criteria

28. In which year was computed tomography made available for clinical practice?

   A   1970
   B   1972
   C   1974
   D   1976
   E   1978

29. Single photon emission computed tomography study in Alzheimer's disease has shown reduced regional blood flow. Which part of the brain is implicated in this?

   A   Anterior parietal area
   B   Cerebellum
   C   Occipital area
   D   Prefrontal area
   E   Posterior parietal area

30. Which of the following statements about Huntington's disease is correct?

   A   Caudate nucleus is not affected
   B   Dopamine concentration is increased in striatum
   C   Extrapyramidal neuronal loss occurs in frontal cortex
   D   γ-Aminobutyric acid concentration is decreased in caudate nucleus
   E   It mainly affects the frontal and temporal lobes

PSYCHOPHARMACOLOGY: PHARMACOKINETICS

31. Which of the statements about the elimination of clonidine is correct?

    A   Clonidine is completely excreted by kidneys unchanged
    B   Clonidine is metabolised completely in the liver before its excretion
    C   Plasma half-life of clonidine is 24 hours
    D   Rate of clonidine metabolism increases with age
    E   Rate of clonidine metabolism is highest in young children under the age of 6

32. Which of the following is consistent with the concept of neurotransmitters?

    A   They are released from the presynaptic terminal when the neuron repolarises
    B   They bind to a receptor, and cause an effect in postsynaptic neurons
    C   The reuptake mechanism can be presynaptic or postsynaptic
    D   They are stored actively in the presynaptic terminal
    E   They are synthesised by presynaptic and postsynaptic neurons

33. What is the rate-limiting step in the synthesis of dopamine?

    A   Catechol-O-methyl transferase
    B   Dopa decarboxylase
    C   Dopamine β-hydroxylase
    D   Phenylalanine hydroxylase
    E   Tyrosine hydroxylase

34. A patient receives an injection of flupenthixol decanoate 50 mg intramuscularly every 2 weeks. In terms of its absorption, what order of kinetics does flupenthixol decanoate follow?

    A   First-order kinetics
    B   Fourth-order kinetics
    C   Second-order kinetics
    D   Third-order kinetics
    E   Zero-order kinetics

35. Which of the following drugs leads to sensitisation?

    A   Alcohol
    B   Amphetamine
    C   Carbamazepine
    D   Diazepam
    E   Heroin

36. Which of the following results in increased excretion of lithium?

    A   Acetazolamide
    B   Aldosterone antagonists
    C K^+-sparing diuretics
    D   Loop diuretics
    E   Thiazide

PSYCHOPHARMACOLOGY: PHARMACODYNAMICS

37. Which of the following pharmacological profiles belongs to bifeprunox?

    A   Binds to D_2-, (5-HT_{2A}-), 5-HT_{2C}-, α_1-/α_2-, low affinity for H_1- and muscarinic receptors

B   Blocks D_1-, D_2- and D_4-receptors and α_1-/α_2-receptors; postural hypotension and hyperprolactinemia are common
C D_1- and D_4-receptor antagonist, 5-HT_{2A}-receptor agonist, strong antihistaminic side effects
D D_2-/5-HT_{2A}-receptor antagonist, little activity at H_1- and muscarinic receptors, insomnia is a common adverse effect
E D_2-receptor partial agonist, 5-HT_{1A}-receptor agonist, low potential for weight gain, extrapyramidal symptoms and hyperprolactinemia

38. Which of the following is the most appropriate strategy for switching from mirtazapine to venlafaxine?

A   Cross-taper cautiously
B   Withdraw mirtazapine and then start venlafaxine
C   Withdraw mirtazapine and wait for 2 weeks before starting venlafaxine
D   Withdraw mirtazapine and wait for 24–48 hours before starting venlafaxine
E   Withdraw mirtazapine and wait for a week before starting venlafaxine

39. Which of the following is a contraindication for sildenafil?

A   Asthma
B   Diabetes
C   Epilepsy
D   Hypertension
E   Myocardial infarction

40. Which of the following statements about differences in the drugs used for dementia is correct?

A   Galantamine decreases the sensitivity of acetylcholine receptors, whereas donepezil and rivastigmine do not
B   Half-lives of donepezil and rivastigmine are about 40 hours and 12 hours respectively
C   Memantine works by protecting neurons from excessive stimulation
D   Rivastigmine and galantamine have less peripheral activity outside the central nervous system than donepezil
E   Rivastigmine is highly protein bound whereas donepezil circulates mostly unbound

41. A 20-year-old man presented with trigeminal neuralgia in the pain clinic. He was prescribed carbamazepine. Which of the following receptors mediate the nociceptic action of carbamazepine?

A   Through γ-aminobutyric acid A (GABA-A) receptor
B   Through GABA-B receptors
C   Through membrane depolarisation
D   Through muscarinic anticholinergic receptor blockade
E   Through central dopaminergic receptors

42. Which of the following is a mechanism of action of galantamine?

A   It acts as a N-methyl-D-aspartate (NMDA) receptor antagonist
B   It is an irreversible inhibitor of anticholinesterase
C   It is a nicotine acetylcholine receptor antagonist
D   It is a NMDA receptor agonist
E   It is a reversible inhibitor of anticholinesterase

43. Which of the following is a mechanism of action of aripiprazole?

A   Antagonist at $(5\text{-}HT_{1A}\text{-})$ receptors
B D_2-receptor antagonism
C D_2-receptor partial agonism
D   Has an anticholinergic effect.
E   Partial agonist at 5-HT_{2A}-receptors

PSYCHOPHARMACOLOGY: ADVERSE REACTIONS

44. A 70-year-old woman taking an antidepressant for the last 3 weeks was admitted to a medical ward following a seizure. This was associated with a history of nausea, dizziness, lethargy, confusion and cramps. Which of the following drugs has been reported the least as being responsible for this presentation?

   A   Citalopram
   B   Clomipramine
   C   Fluoxetine
   D   Moclobemide
   E   Venlafaxine

45. Which of the following is most likely to develop earlier in the course of serotonin syndrome rather than late?

   A   Blood pressure instability
   B   Diarrhoea
   C   Hyperreflexia
   D   Myoclonus
   E   Rigidity

46. A 34-year-old woman on lithium for about 5 years presented to her general practitioner with adverse effects. Which of the following is suggestive of lithium toxicity?

   A   Coarse tremors
   B   Diarrhoea
   C   Nephrogenic diabetes insipidus
   D   Rashes
   E   Renal tubular acidosis

47. What is the mechanism of sedation caused by clonidine?

   A   Imidazoline receptor antagonism
   B   Postsynaptic α_2-adrenoreceptor agonism
   C   Postsynaptic α_1-adrenoreceptor agonism
   D   Presynaptic α_1-adrenoreceptor agonism
   E   Presynaptic α_2-adrenoreceptor agonism

48. Which of the following drugs causes hyperprolactinemia?

   A   Aripiprazole
   B   Diazepam
   C   Fluoxetine
   D   Lithium
   E   Mirtazapine

49. Which of the following can result in postinjection delirium/sedation syndrome?

   A   Flupenthixol decanoate
   B   Haloperidol decanoate
   C   Olanzapine pamoate
   D   Paliperidone palmitate
   E   Risperdal Consta

50. Which of the following is a dose-related side effect?

   A   Clozapine-induced agranulocytosis
   B   Clozapine-induced deep vein thrombosis

    C   Clozapine-induced diabetes mellitus
    D   Clozapine-induced myocarditis
    E   Clozapine-related seizures

51. Which of the following side effects of antipsychotics is not dose dependent?

    A   Extrapyramidal side effects
    B   Neuroleptic malignant syndrome
    C   Postural hypotension
    D   QTc prolongation
    E   Sudden cardiac death

52. A 23-year-old man with schizophrenia was treated with antipsychotic medication. He complained of breast discharge and loss of libido. Which of the following antipsychotics should be used as an alternative option?

    A   Amisulpride
    B   Chlorpromazine
    C   Haloperidol
    D   Olanzapine
    E   Risperidone

PSYCHOPHARMACOLOGY: THEORIES OF ACTION

53. Which of the following drugs is least effective as a prophylactic agent for bipolar affective disorder?

    A   Aripiprazole
    B   Clozapine
    C   Lamotrigine
    D   Olanzapine
    E   Topiramate

54. What is the fortnightly maintenance dose of olanzapine pamoate injection after 2 months of treatment for a patient taking 15 mg olanzapine?

    A   100 mg
    B   150 mg
    C   210 mg
    D   300 mg
    E   405 mg

55. A 55-year-old man was referred by the cardiologist for assessment of his depression. He has had a myocardial infarction (MI) recently. Which antidepressant has the best evidence base for its use in post-MI depression?

    A   Amitriptyline
    B   Citalopram
    C   Fluoxetine
    D   Reboxetine
    E   Sertraline

56. A 30-year-old man diagnosed with schizophrenia was treated with three different antipsychotics for about 6 months at therapeutic doses without any significant improvement. He was started on clozapine recently. What are the chances that his condition will respond to clozapine?

    A   10%
    B   20%

C   30%
D   40%
E   50%

PSYCHOPHARMACOLOGY: DRUG DEPENDENCE

57. A drug causes release of catecholamines as well as serotonin. This drug is taken up in serotoninergic neurons by the serotonin transporter responsible for 5-hydroxytryptamine (5-HT) reuptake and, once inside the neuron, it causes rapid release of a bolus of 5-HT. What is this drug called?

A   Amphetamine
B   Cannabis
C   Cocaine
D   Ecstasy
E   Lysergic acid diethylamide

PSYCHOPHARMACOLOGY: NEW DRUGS

58. Which of the following statement applies to varenicline?

A   It is available as injection
B   It is indicated for the treatment of opioid dependence
C   It is recommended to be used for 6 weeks in one course of treatment
D   It is a D_2-receptor partial agonist
E   Its use can precipitate or exacerbate psychosis

GENETICS: CELLULAR AND MOLECULAR GENETICS

59. Which of the following will demonstrate fragile sites in chromosomes?

A   Cell culture devoid of pyrimidine
B   Culturing cells in conditions devoid of thymidine
C   Culturing cells in medium devoid of folate
D   Culturing cells in medium devoid of vitamin B_{12}
E   Karyotyping

60. Which of the following statements about the structure of DNA is correct?

A   Its back bone is made of two chains of sugars wrapped in the form of double helix, held together by hydrogen bonds
B   Its backbone is made from alternating phosphate and sugar residues, held together by hydrogen bonds
C   It has two chains of nucleotides wrapped in the form of a double helix, held together by ester bonds
D   It has two chains of nucleotides wrapped in the form of a double helix, held together by hydrogen bonds
E   It has two chains of nucleotides wrapped in the form of a double helix, held together by covalent bonds

61. Of what is the basic repeat unit of DNA made?

   A   Deoxyribose sugar, a carbon group and a nitrogenous base
   B   Deoxyribose sugar and a nitrogenous base
   C   Deoxyribose sugar and a phosphate group
   D   Deoxyribose sugar, nitrogenous base and a carbon group
   E   Deoxyribose sugar, nitrogenous base and a phosphate group

62. Which of the following cell organelles is essential for translation or decoding?

   A   Endoplasmic reticulum
   B   Mitochondrion
   C   Nucleolus
   D   Nucleus
   E   Ribosome

63. Which of the following statements about mitosis is correct?

   A   It contains only one of each pair of chromosomes
   B   It is described as diploid
   C   It is described as haploid
   D   It forms gametes
   E   It means segregation of parent cells

64. Which of the following statements about the frame-shift mutation responsible for Tay–Sachs disease is correct?

   A   There is breakage of a fragment of chromosome and re-joining at a different site
   B   A piece of DNA is gained
   C   There is a simple change in one base of the gene sequence due to substitution of one base by another
   D   There is a loss of one base, causing the triplet code to be read out of the frame
   E   There is a loss in the sequence of bases

65. Which of the following statements about restriction enzymes found mainly in bacteria is correct?

   A   They act by cutting DNA randomly
   B   They are also called restriction methyltransferases
   C   They are mainly used for modification of RNA in the laboratory settings
   D   They can be used to get fragments of easily manageable base-pair sizes (10^3–10^4), thus allowing genes to be handled almost in isolation
   E   They are used by bacteria for the synthesis of bacterial protein

66. Which of the following statements about reverse transcriptase is correct?

   A   It is a restriction enzyme
   B   It is used in synthesis of complementary DNA from mRNA
   C   It is used to break down tRNA into different segments
   D   It is used to stop the synthesis of a defective protein in humans
   E   It reverses the process of transcription in a cell, thus halting the production of an abnormal base sequence

67. Denaturing gradient gel electrophoresis, chemical cleavage, single-strand conformational analysis and heteroduplex analysis are used for identification of causal mutations. What is the basis of this process?

   A   DNA sequencing
   B   Northern blotting

C   Polymerase chain reaction
D   Southern blotting
E   Western blotting

68. Which of the following statements about restriction fragment length polymorphism analysis is correct?

A   It is detected by south-western blotting
B   It is generally inherited in a non-mendelian fashion
C   It is an important component of positional cloning
D   It is based on the fact that DNA fragments produced by digestion by a certain restriction enzyme will be of different lengths in different individuals
E   It is based on the fact that DNA fragments produced by digestion by a certain restriction enzyme will be same lengths in different individuals because they cleave at a specific base sequence site

69. To what does genetics imprinting lead?

A   Change in the sequence of DNA
B   Duplication of DNA
C   Irreversible gene inactivation
D   Mutation of a gene
E   Reversible gene inactivation

GENETICS: BEHAVIOURAL GENETICS

70. Which are the commonest association studies in psychiatric literature?

A   Allelic association studies
B   Candidate gene association studies
C   Multiple testing studies
D   Population stratification studies
E   Whole genome association studies

71. What is the heritability of antisocial behaviour?

A   20%
B   30%
C   40%
D   50%
E   60%

72. To date, which condition has the strongest evidence for gene and environment interaction?

A   Antisocial behaviour
B   Bipolar affective disorder
C   Borderline personality disorder
D   Depression
E   Schizophrenia

73. Which of the following metabolic diseases has X-linked transmission?

A   Gaucher's disease
B   Hunter's syndrome
C   Hurler's syndrome

D   Marquio's syndrome
E   Metachromatic leukodystrophy

74. When we consider linkage studies with heterogeneity, what does 'allelic heterogeneity' mean?

A   The cases are either polygenic in inheritance or not genetic at all
B   Two or more loci at which an allelic mutation occurs result in different phenotype
C   Two or more mutant alleles existing at different loci result in same phenotypes
D   Two or more mutant alleles existing at same locus result in same phenotypes
E   Two or more mutant alleles existing at same locus result in different phenotypes

75. What does the term 'vertical inheritance' in genetics mean?

A   Transmission of disease from mother to offspring
B   Transmission of disease from father to offspring
C   The phenomenon that affected individuals is found in every generation
D   The phenomenon that affected invividuals is seen every second generation
E   No cases may occur in a previous generation, and the disease may manifest in children of the next generation

76. In neurofibromatosis, some patients may have only café-au-lait spots, whereas others may have more features including neurofibromas, café-au-lait spots. What is the phenomenon called in which there is manifestation of symptoms of variable degree in different individuals with the same genotype?

A   Dominance
B   Expressivity
C   Manifestation
D   Penetrance
E   Visibility

77. Which of the RNA polymerases is involved in protein synthesis in humans?

A   RNA polymerase I
B   RNA Polymerase II
C   RNA polymerase III
D   RNA polymerase IV
E   RNA polymerase V

GENETICS: ENDOPHENOTYPES

78. Which of the following disturbs the Hardy–Weinberg equilibrium?

A   A population that does not allow migrated communities to mix with them
B   Marriages among close relatives not allowed
C   No changes in gene frequencies because of a chance factor
D   No mutations in a population
E   Mating among professionals with a high IQ

79. Which of the following is an endophenotype related to sensory gating deficits in schizophrenia?

A   Ambivalence
B   Circumstantiality
C   Impulsivity
D   Prepulse inhibition
E   Pseudohallucinations

80. Which of the following genes is implicated in the transport of amyloid precursor protein to endoplasmic reticulum for degradation?

    A   Amyloid precursor protein gene
    B   Apolipoprotein E44
    C   Presenilin 2
    D   Presenilin1
    E   Sortilin-related receptor (*SORL1*) gene

GENETICS: GENETIC EPIDEMIOLOGY

81. What is the concordance rate of schizophrenia in dizygotic twins?

    A   5%
    B   14%
    C   30%
    D   46%
    E   85%

82. Smoking cannabis at young age increases the risk of developing schizophrenia. Which of the concepts explains this association?

    A   Cofactor
    B   Dominant
    C   Epithetic
    D   Epigenetics
    E   Epistasis

83. What is the prevalence of 22Q deletion syndrome in patients with schizophrenia?

    A   0.5%
    B   1%
    C   5%
    D   10%
    E   15%

84. A 45-year-old man with choreiform movements presented in the neuropsychiatric clinic. He was diagnosed with Huntington's disease. Genetic testing showed that he had the Huntingtin gene in only one of the chromosomes (C4). His wife did not have Huntington's disease. He wanted to know the chances of his son developing the disorder. What would you say to him?

    A   100%
    B   50%
    C   25%
    D   10%
    E   1%

GENETICS: GENE–ENVIRONMENT INTERACTION

85. Which of the following describes path analysis correctly?

    A   Analyse the path of a patient through the services
    B   Analysis of biochemical pathways in the brain of mentally disordered individuals
    C   Analysis of evolution of symptoms in a mentally disordered individual

D Analysis of the gene–environment interaction using biological techniques
E Analysis of the gene–environment interaction using statistical techniques

86. What is the unit of measurement of genetic distance?

A Centilitres
B Centimorgans
C Centimetres
D Kilobases
E Ounces

87. Which of the following statements is the most accurate definition of a recombination fraction?

A It is defined as the fraction of genes that cross-over
B It is defined as the number of recombinants divided by the total number of offsprings
C It is defined as the total number of offspring divided by the number of recombinants
D It is defined as the total number of recombinants divided by the number of recombinants
E It is defined as the total number of recombinants divided by the number of non-recombinants

88. You analysed the genome of a person to find the genetic marker for Huntington's disease. For him to be negative for the genetic marker, what should the logarithm of odds score be?

A −2
B −1
C 0
D 1
E 2

89. What is the genotypic correlation between two siblings?

A 0.1
B 0.25
C 0.5
D 0.75
E 1

90. Which of the following statements about schizotaxia is correct?

A It is ataxia in a patient with schizophrenia
B It is a catatonic sign
C It is a form of thought disorder seen in patients with schizophrenia
D It is a form of thought disorder seen in schizotypal personality disorder
E It is a liability to develop schizophrenia from childhood

EPIDEMIOLOGY: SURVEYS ACROSS THE LIFESPAN

91. What type of study would you consider if you want to understand why some people cope with a chronic illness well, whereas others find it difficult to cope?

A Case–control study
B Cohort study
C Cross-sectional survey
D Qualitative study
E Randomised controlled study

92. Which of the following statements about a confounder is correct?

    A   It is a variable that is present on the casual pathway between the exposure and the outcome
    B   It cannot be reduced by restricting the study population
    C   It varies systematically with an exposure and acts as an independent risk or protective factor for the disease
    D   It is a variable introduced to minimise the biases in the study
    E   It should not be in a triangular relationship with the other variables

93. Which of the following is the most common psychiatric disorder in primary care?

    A   Anxiety disorder
    B   Depression
    C   Generalised anxiety disorder
    D   Mixed anxiety and depressive disorder
    E   Panic attacks

94. Which of the following is associated with twice the risk of developing a neurotic disorder amongst the general population?

    A   Belonging to a lower social class
    B   No qualification
    C   Prisoner and homeless
    D   Unemployed person
    E   Urban living

95 How common are specific phobias in the general population?

    A   2%
    B   2.5%
    C   10%
    D   5%
    E   20%

96. An audit of suicides in 5000 depressed patients in a population found that 100 patients had taken their own life. The rate of suicide therefore was 100/5000. What does this rate refer to?

    A   Case fatality rate
    B   Cause-specific mortality rate
    C   Crude mortality rate
    D   Proportional mortality rate
    E   Specific mortality rate

97. Which of the following statements about variant Creutzfeldt-Jakob disease (vCJD) is correct when compared with CJD?

    A   EEG abnormalities are less common in variant CJD
    B   The 'pulvinar sign' on MRI is not a diagnostic sign in variant CJD
    C   Variant CJD has a delayed onset
    D   Variant CJD has a rapid course
    E   Variant CJD rarely presents with psychiatric features such as depression and personality changes

98. What is the percentage of the transvestites who are diagnosed as having a personality disorder?

    A   10–30%
    B   30–50%
    C   50–70%
    D   70–90%
    E   90–99%

99. In which age group does three-quarters of life-time mental illness occur?

    A   Mid-20s
    B   Mid-30s
    C   Mid-40s
    D   Mid-50s
    E   Mid-60s

100. Evidence suggested that the rate of suicide had increased manyfold in women who were imprisoned. What is the likely increase?

    A   5
    B   10
    C   15
    D   20
    E   25

101. What percentage of people with mental illness consume tobacco in the UK?

    A   30%
    B   40%
    C   50%
    D   60%
    E   70%

102. Which of the following statements about head injury is correct?

    A   Children are at greater risk from 5–15 years of age
    B   On average 1000/100,0000 attend hospital with a head injury every year
    C   Only 50% of the head injuries are severe
    D   Risk factors include higher socioeconomic class
    E   Road traffic accidents are the commonest cause of head injury

103. Which of the following statements about the association of immigration with schizophrenia is correct?

    A   Risk is higher in second-generation migrants than first-generation migrants
    B   Risk is higher for first-generation migrants than second-generation migrants
    C   Risk is higher for migrants from higher socioeconomic status
    D   Risk is higher for white people moving into black societies
    E   Risk is increased in the parents but not the siblings of the second generation

104. A spurious association in an ecological study found at population level did not hold at an individual level. What is this called?

    A   Ceiling effect
    B   Central limit theorem
    C   Ecological fallacy
    D   Halo effect
    E   Hawthorne effect

EPIDEMIOLOGY: MEASURES

105. A town in the UK has a population of 90,000. There were 1000 and 1100 patients in 2009 and 2010, respectively, diagnosed with benign melanoma. What was the incidence rate of the disease in 2010 among the town population?

    A   1000/90,000

B   1200/90,000
C   1100/89,000
D   1200/89,000
E   2000/90,000

106. In the above question what was the prevalence in 2010?

A   1000/90,000
B   1200/90,000
C   1000/89,000
D   1100/89,000
E   2100/90,000

107. In a city, the incidence of schizophrenia among people using cannabis was 80/1000 whereas the incidence in those people who did not use cannabis was 20/1000. What is the relative risk of developing schizophrenia in this population?

A   2
B   4
C   6
D   8
E   10

108. In the above question what would be the attribution risk?

A   20
B   40
C   60
D   80
E   100

109. On the global assessment scale, what is the score for the severe range of symptoms?

A   0–10
B   21–30
C   41–50
D   71–80
E   91–100

110. Which test is most useful in confirming cerebral dominance before planning destructive brain surgery?

A   Electrophysiological testing
B   Halstead–Reitan neuropsychological battery
C   Repeatable battery for assessment of neuropsychological status
D   Wada test
E   Word association test

111. What does an asymmetrical funnel plot indicate?

A   Arbitrary
B   Confounding
C   Inference
D   Publication bias
E   Recruitment bias

112. Survival times are thought not to obey a normal distribution. Which of the following measures is used?

A   Forest plot

B   Hazard ratio
C   Kaplan–Meier curve
D   Linear curve
E   River plot

ADVANCED PSYCHOLOGICAL PROCESSES AND TREATMENTS: PERSONALITY AND PERSONALITY DISORDER

113. Which of the following is one of the big five personality factors?

A   Aggressive
B   Decisiveness
C   Introversion
D   Neuroticism
E   Psychoticism

114. Which of the following factors is associated with higher rates of inpatient admissions in patients with borderline personality disorder?

A   Anxiety disorders
B   Depressive disorders
C   Psychotic disorders
D   Severity of para-suicides
E   Substance misuse

115. With regard to the cost of treatment for people with borderline personality disorder, which of the following statements is correct?

A   Regular hospital treatment for borderline personality disorder is no more expensive than treatment as usual, and shows considerable cost savings after treatment
B   Specialist full hospital treatment for borderline personality disorder is no more expensive than treatment as usual, and shows considerable cost savings after treatment
C   Specialist partial hospital treatment for borderline personality disorder is no more expensive than treatment as usual, and shows considerable cost savings after treatment
D   Specialist partial hospital treatment for borderline personality disorder is more expensive than treatment as usual, and shows considerable cost savings after treatment
E   Specialist partial hospital treatment for borderline personality disorder is no more expensive than treatment as usual, and does not show considerable cost savings after treatment

116. Which of the following is effective in the treatment of schizotypal personality disorder?

A   Anticonvulsant drug
B   Antidepressant drug
C   Antipsychotic drug
D   Benzodiazepines
E   Mood stabilisers

117. As far as the evidence for psychological therapies in borderline personality disorder is concerned, which of the following statements is correct?

A   Cognitive–behavioural therapy should be considered if reducing self-harm is a priority
B   Convincing evidence from randomised controlled trials shows that the individual psychological therapies are effective
C   Dialectical behavioural therapy is ineffective in reducing self-harm in women

    D   Evidence base for psychological therapies in the treatment of borderline personality disorder is good

    E   Mentalisation-based therapy with partial hospitalisation is effective in reducing suicide attempts and self-harm

ADVANCED PSYCHOLOGICAL PROCESSES AND TREATMENTS: DEVELOPMENTAL PSYCHOPATHOLOGY (INCLUDING TEMPERAMENT)

118. Which of the following correctly defines one of the needs according to Maslow's hierarchy of needs?

    A   Aesthetic: understanding

    B   Belonging: recognition

    C   Physiological: absence of danger

    D   Self-actualisation: knowledge

    E   Self-esteem: social acceptance

119. Which of the following parenting styles results in children who are happy, capable and successful adults?

    A   Authoritarian

    B   Authoritative

    C   Good-enough parent

    D   Neglectful

    E   Permissive

120. What is the most likely effect on a child whose mother has a history of depression?

    A   Child has normal behaviour

    B   Child can develop depression in later life

    C   Child has easy temperament

    D   Cognitive functioning is usually higher

    E   Stable attachments are formed

121. With regard to effects of maternal mental illness on infants, which of the following statements is correct?

    A   Bipolar affective disorder has devastating effects on an infant

    B   Depressed mothers develop better relationships with the infants

    C   If identified and treated early, puerperal psychosis is relatively benign

    D   Manic episodes have a devastating effect on relationships with the infants

    E   Postnatal depressive illness does not cause behavioural disturbances in infants

122. Which of the following is considered as an explanatory model for mothers acting as an agent for the development of child psychopathology?

    A   Attachment relationship is secure

    B   Children of mothers with postnatal depression have no continuing disadvantages

    C   General parenting is unaffected

    D   Postnatal depression is more apparent in children coming from deprived backgrounds

    E   Serious consequences for the children do not occur as a result of maternal mental illness

123. Which of the following is considered an explanatory model for the child to act as an agent in the development of psychopathology in the mother?

A   Affection from child
B   Childbirth unrelated
C   Children having no impact on marital intimacy
D   Children with difficult temperaments being less likely to have depressed mothers
E   Ill or disabled children

124. Who proposed the strange situation test?

A   Ainsworth
B   Bowlby
C   Harlow
D   Main
E   Rutter

125. Which of the following statements describes the concept of goodness of fit most accurately?

A   A child should be easy, active and sociable
B   Difficult temperament is maladaptive
C   Mother does not have to be perfect, but good enough
D   Negative developments arise in a child when the temperament and environment match
E   There are reciprocal relations hips between a baby and the environment

126. Which of the following concepts was proposed by Bowlby?

A   Cognitive behaviourism and social learning
B   Inner working models of attachment
C   Self-perception theory
D   Theory of hedonism
E   Theory of motivation

127. Which of the following is an important contribution of Carl Jung to the field of psychoanalysis?

A   Depressive position
B   Internal objects
C   Paranoid–schizoid position
D   Projective identification
E   Shadow

ADVANCED PSYCHOLOGICAL PROCESSES AND TREATMENTS: THERAPY MODELS, METHODS, PROCESSES AND OUTCOMES

128. Which of the following theories was proposed by Freud?

A   Attachment and effects of early experiences
B   Evolution of adult consciousness
C   Restoration theory of sleep
D   Theory of adult consciousness
E   Theory of hedonism

129. Which of the following statements about reinforcement is correct?

   A   Being paid monthly is an example of fixed-ratio reinforcement
   B   Commissioning is a type of continuous reinforcement
   C   Extinction occurs rapidly in variable-interval reinforcement
   D   Gambling is an example of variable-ratio reinforcement
   E   Resistance to extinction is high in continuous reinforcement

130. Which of the following mechanisms takes place in dreams?

   A   Altruism
   B   Denial
   C   Displacement
   D   Projection
   E   Sublimation

131. Which of the following is used in providing an incentive as part of contingency management in patients who misuse drugs?

   A   Clinic privileges
   B   Family-based reinforcement
   C   Friend-based reinforcement
   D   Home-based reinforcement
   E   School-based reinforcement

132. According to the current evidence, which of the following statements about psychological therapies in drug misuse is correct?

   A   Contingency management is associated with continuous periods of abstinence in cocaine misuse
   B   Couple-based behavioural therapy is used where both partners are misusing drugs
   C   Relapse prevention has been found to be an effective treatment for cocaine dependence
   D   Relapse prevention has been found to be an effective treatment for heroin dependence
   E   Social systems interventions were developed primarily for elderly people misusing drugs

133. According to the current evidence, which of the following statements about psychological therapies delivered in the outpatient settings for anorexia nervosa is correct?

   A   Cognitive–behavioural therapy (CBT) is more acceptable to patients than dietary counselling after weight restoration in hospital
   B   One of the aims of therapy is to prevent deliberate self-harm and suicide attempts
   C   There is good evidence that family interventions at tertiary centres are superior to 'treatment as usual'
   D   There is good evidence that family intervention is superior to interpersonal therapy by the end of treatment
   E   There is limited evidence that individual supportive psychotherapy is superior to family therapy in terms of weight gain

134. According to the current evidence, which of the following is an effective psychological therapy for the treatment of anorexia nervosa?

   A   CBT–bulimia nervosa
   B   Exposure and response prevention
   C   Focal psychodynamic psychotherapy
   D   Guided self-help
   E   Simplified dialectical behaviour therapy

135. According to current evidence, which of the following statements about psychological therapies in bulimia nervosa is correct?

    A   Cognitive behavioural therapy–bulimia nervosa (CBT-BN) is more acceptable to patients than interpersonal therapy–bulimia nervosa (IPT-BN), psychodynamic psychotherapy or dietary counselling

    B   CBT-BN is superior to dietary counselling for managing purging by the end of treatment

    C   CBT-BN is superior to dietary counselling for managing purging by the end of follow-up

    D   IPT-BN is superior to CBT-BN in terms of remission from binge eating

    E   IPT-BN is superior to CBT-BN in terms of remission from purging

136. According to the current evidence, which of the following statements about psychological therapies for treating depression is correct?

    A   Ten to twelve sessions of CBT are sufficient for most patients to achieve lasting remission

    B   Sixteen to twenty sessions of both psychodynamic psychotherapy and CBT are insufficient for most patients to achieve lasting remission

    C   Sixteen to twenty sessions of psychodynamic psychotherapy are sufficient for most patients to achieve lasting remission

    D   CBT is superior to short-term psychodynamic psychotherapy in improving social functioning

    E   CBT is superior to short-term psychodynamic psychotherapy in treating depressive symptoms

137. According to the current evidence, which of the following statements about delivery of psychological therapies to patients is correct?

    A   CBT research has focused on the development and mechanism of action rather than evaluating treatment programmes

    B   For more complex interventions, therapists require longer training to be competent therapists

    C   Guided self-help without seeing a skilled therapist in post-traumatic stress disorder has outcomes similar to those when a therapist is available

    D   Self-study-assisted CBT with a few individual sessions is inferior to full CBT

    E   Therapist's personal attributes and styles are more important than therapist training

138. According to current evidence, which of the following statements about psychotherapy for patients with depression or dysthymia is correct?

    A   Sixteen to twenty sessions of psychotherapy are required for the optimal effects of psychotherapy

    B   Combined treatment is better than psychotherapy alone but equal in efficacy compared with pharmacotherapy

    C   Psychotherapy is almost as effective as pharmacotherapy for depressed patients

    D   Psychotherapy is as good as pharmacotherapy for dysthymic patients

    E   Psychotherapy is better than pharmacotherapy for dysthymic patients

139. Which of the following statements about 'linking' is correct?

    A   It is a behavioural experience that establishes the nature of a relationship between phenomena or objects

    B   It is a cognitive process that establishes the nature of a relationship between phenomena or objects

    C   It is an emotional experience that establishes the nature of a relationship between phenomena or objects

    D   It is a thought process that establishes the nature of a relationship between phenomena or objects

    E   It is a connection between the attachment figure and the child

140. Which of the following is considered as the most effective treatment for binge eating disorder?

    A   Behavioural weight loss
    B   Behavioural weight loss + CBT
    C   CBT
    D   Supportive psychotherapy
    E   Treatment as usual

141. Which of the following statements about NICE (National Institute for Health and Care Excellence) guidelines for psychological treatment of generalised anxiety disorder is correct?

    A   Applied relaxation is an ineffective treatment compared with wait list control
    B   CBT was not found to be an effective treatment compared with wait list control
    C   CBT was found to be neither inferior nor superior to applied relaxation
    D   No evidence showed that CBT is more effective than psychodynamic therapy
    E   No evidence showed that CBT is effective in short-term management

Answers: MCQs

1. B Hypothalamus

This develops as a part of the limbic system, which is concerned with preservation of the individual and of the species. In the sagittal plane, the hypothalamus is divided into three regions: anterior, middle and posterior. Mammillary nuclei are part of the posterior region. Basal ganglia are associated with the control of movements. It includes striatum (caudate nucleus, putamen of lentiform nucleus, nucleus accumbens), pallidum (global pallidus of lentiform nucleus) which has medial and lateral segments, the subthalamic nucleus and the pigmented part of the substantia nigra.

2. D Mammillary body

The thalamus is the largest nuclear mass in the entire nervous system. The posterior part of the ventral lateral nucleus, ventral anterior, medial geniculate body, anterior thalamic nucleus and lateral geniculate body supply afferents to the cerebellum, globus pallidus, inferior colliculus, mammillary body and superior colliculus, respectively.

3. E Ipsilateral scotoma

Deficits at different locations in the visual pathway lead to different visual field defects. Scotoma is an area of partial or complete blindness that is surrounded by near normal vision. A lesion in a part of the optic nerve leads to ipsilateral scotoma, whereas a partial lesion in the bilateral optic nerve leads to bilateral scotoma. A lesion in the complete optic nerve leads to blindness in the ipsilateral eye. A lesion in the optic chiasma leads to bitemporal hemianopia. A lesion in the optic tract leads to homonymous hemianopia. A lesion in Meyer's loop leads to homonymous upper quadrantanopia. A lesion in the optic radiation and visual cortex leads to homonymous hemianopia. A lesion in the bilateral macular cortex leads to bilateral central scotomas.

4. B Meyer's loop

This is a part of the optic radiation on the visual pathway. Damage in the temporal lobe, resulting in a lesion in Meyer's loop, leads to homonymous upper quadrantanopia. Homonymous hemianopia with macular sparing can occur due to posterior cerebral ischaemia and migraine.

5. B Frontal operculum

The frontal lobe consists of the frontal operculum, superior and inferior mesial regions, and dorsolateral prefrontal cortex. The frontal operculum consists of Brodmann's areas 44, 45 and 47. Broca's areas (44 and 45) are located in the dominant hemisphere of the brain.

6. B Diencephalon

Primary brain vesicles are divided into the prosencephalon, mesencephalon and rhombencephalon. The prosencephalon is further divided into the telencephalon and diencephalon. The telencephalon gives rise to the cerebral hemisphere and parts of the basal ganglia. The diencephalon gives rise to the thalamus, hypothalamus, posterior pituitary, optic nerve and retina. The mesencephalon gives rise to the midbrain. The rhombencephalon is divided into the metencephalon, which gives rise to the pons and cerebellum, and the myelencephalon, which gives rise to the medulla oblongata.

7. C Inferior mesial region

The frontal lobe consists of the frontal operculum, superior mesial region, inferior mesial region and dorsolateral prefrontal cortex. The inferior mesial region consists of orbital cortex and basal forebrain. The frontal operculum consists of areas 44, 45 and 47. The superior mesial region consists of the supplementary motor area and anterior cingulate cortex.

8. E Vestibulocochlear nerve

In total, there are 12 cranial nerves. The eighth cranial nerve is called the vestibulocochlear nerve. It consists of two parts, namely vestibular and cochlear. The cochlear nerve fibres terminate in anterior and posterior cochlear nuclei.

9. B Cingulate gyrus

The limbic lobe is an arrangement of cortical structures around the diencephalon. It consists of cortical areas and nuclei. The cortical areas include the cingulate gyrus, parahippocampal gyrus and subcallosal gyrus. Its nuclei include the amygdaloid nucleus and septal nucleus. The hypothalamus, olfactory bulb, amygdala, and septal and some thalamic nuclei are part of the subcortical portion of the limbic system.

10. A Bilateral acoustic neurofibromatosis

The prevalence of bilateral acoustic neurofibromatosis is 1/106. Its clinicopathological features are multiple intracranial and spinal tumours, mainly schwannomas and neurofibromas. Tuberous sclerosis has clinicopathological features such as cutaneous lesions consisting of shagreen patch, subungual angiofibromas, glial nodes in the cortex and adjacent to ventricle, rhabdomyomas of the heart, learning disability and epilepsy. The Sturge–Webber syndrome consists of a strawberry naevus/port wine stain on face, angiomatous malformation of meningeal vessels with calcification, along with learning disability and epilepsy. The von Hippel–Lindau disease is rare and has vascular malformation of the retina, haemangioblastoma and pancreatic, adrenal and renal cysts and tumours.

11. C Pick's bodies

The macroscopic changes seen in Alzheimer's disease are global brain atrophy, ventricular enlargement and sulcal widening. These changes are mostly seen in the frontal and temporal lobes. The macroscopic changes seen in Pick's disease are selective asymmetrical atrophy of anterior frontal and temporal lobes, knife blade gyri and ventricular enlargement. The histological changes seen in Pick's disease include Pick's bodies, neuronal loss and reactive astrocytosis.

12. A Arteriosclerotic changes in major arteries

Macroscopic changes seen in multi-infarct dementia are multiple cerebral infarcts, local and general brain atrophy, ventricular enlargement and arteriosclerotic changes in major arteries. Sulcal widening is mainly seen in Alzheimer's dementia. Histological changes including infarction and ischaemia are seen in multi-infarct dementia.

13. C Local or general brain atrophy

Histological changes including infarction and ischaemia are seen in multi-infarct dementia and histopathological changes seen in Lewy body dementia include the presence of Lewy bodies, neuronal loss, neurofibrillary tangles and neuritic plaques.

14. C Medulloblastomas

The following cerebral tumours are arranged in the relative frequency of occurrence: gliomas, metastases, meningeal and pituitary tumours, adenomas, neurilemmomas, haemangioblastomas and medulloblastomas. Medulloblastomas are cerebellar tumours, which are embryonal tumours.

15. B Amyloid plaques containing prion protein (PrP)

Prion diseases can be inherited, or acquired infectiously or iatrogenically, although some cases are sporadic. Prion diseases are caused by a proteinacious infectious particle called a 'prion'. 'Prion protein' (PrP) is encoded by a gene on chromosome 20. Normal PrP is denoted as 'PrPc' and when PrPc takes an abnormal conformation, causing prion disease, it is denoted as PrPsc (named after scrapie, the prion disease that affects sheep). The amyloid plaques contain PrP protein and not β-amyloid which is found in Alzheimer's disease. Common neuropathological features are diffuse spongiosis, neuronal loss, gliosis and amyloid plaques containing PrP.

16. D Prolactin

Dopamine has a direct effect on the lactotrophs. They bind to D_2-receptors and inhibit both the synthesis and the secretion of prolactin. All antipsychotic medication can affect the prolactin level.

17. E Somatostatin

Dopamine and somatostatin are inhibitory hypothalamic hormones; arginine vasopressin, corticotrophin-releasing hormone, gonadotrophin-releasing hormone and growth hormone-releasing hormone are stimulating hypothalamic hormones.

18. D α1

Receptors such as μ, δ, κ, cholecystokinin (CCK-A), CCK-B, corticotrophin-releasing hormone and thyrotrophin-releasing hormone are associated with slow transmitters such as opioid-type enkephalin, β-endorphins, dynorphins, cholecystokinin, corticotrophin-releasing hormone and thyrotrophin-releasing hormone respectively. The α_1- and α_2-receptors are associated with a moderate second messenger-linked noradrenaline transmitters.

19. B Ib

As per the Lloyd–Hunt classification of nerve fibres:

Ia – muscle spindle afferents

Ib – tendon organs

II – cutaneous mechanoreceptor

III – deep pressure sensors in muscle

IV – unmyelinated pain fibres.

20. E Influx of sodium into the cell leads to depolarisation

A change in sodium permeability is responsible for initiation of the action potential. On depolarisation, the voltage-gated sodium channels open and there is an influx of sodium into the cell. During the action potential, the neuronal membrane cannot be stimulated and is said to be in a refractory period. On repolarisation, the voltage-gated sodium channels close and the potassium channels open. The action potential leads to depolarisation of adjacent membrane without decrement. However, the speed is dependent on the resistance and capacitance of the membrane, e.g. myelinated and unmyelinated membranes.

21. E Somatostatin

A neurohormone is a chemical that is released by neuroendocrine cells of the hypothalamus and acts at a specific distant site or sites. β-Endorphin and cortisol are not neurohormones. β-Endorphin is an endogenous opioid peptide neurotransmitter. Cortisol is a steroid hormone secreted by the adrenal gland.

It stimulates hormone secretion as follows:

Table 4.1 Neurohormones

Neurohormone	In hypothalamus produced by following neuroendocrine cells	Hormone
Arginine vasopressin or antidiuretic hormone Corticotrophin-releasing hormone	Magnocellular cells Parvocellular cells	Stimulate adrenocorticotrophic hormone
Oxytocin	Magnocellular cells	Stimulate prolactin
Somatostatin	Periventricular nucleus cells	Inhibit growth hormone
Growth hormone-releasing hormone	Arcuate nucleus neurons	Stimulate growth hormone
Gonadotrophin-releasing hormone	Preoptic area cells	Stimulate follicle-stimulating hormone
Thyrotrophin-releasing hormone	Parvocellular cells	Stimulate thyroid-stimulating hormone Stimulate follicle-stimulating hormone

22. A Choline

As far as precursors is concerned choline and acetyl-coenzyme A are precursors of acetylcholine. L-Tyrosine, L-dopa and dopamine are precursors of noradrenaline. L-Tryptophan is the precursor of serotonin. L-Tyrosine and L-dopa are precursors of dopamine and histidine is the precursor of histamine.

23. B Ligand-gated ion channel

Transmembrane receptors are of two types: ionotrophic and metabotrophic receptors.

Ionotrophic receptors are also called ligand-gated ion channel receptors, such as nicotinic cholinergic, γ-aminobutyric acid (GABA-A), glycine and glutamate. These receptors control ion channels directly. Metabotrophic receptors are linked to G-protein-coupled receptors and act indirectly on ion channels via enzymes/second messengers, e.g. GABA-B, visual pigments, and adrenergic and serotoninergic receptors. Membrane-bound receptors similar to G-protein are tyrosine kinase-linked receptors, e.g. neurotrophins, nerve growth factor, brain-derived neurotrophic factor. Steroid- and thyroid-like receptors are intracellular receptors.

24. C Increased β-adrenoreceptors in cortical area

The following changes have been identified in patients with depression:

Increased 5-hydroxytryptamine in limbic area.

Increased muscarinic receptors in limbic area.

Increased β-adrenoreceptors in cortical area.

Decreased 5-HIAA in several regions of the brain and the cerebrospinal fluid.

There is no identified change noticed in nicotinic receptors.

These changes also indicate the mechanism of action of antidepressant medications.

25. C L-Tyrosine

As far as precursors are concerned choline and acetyl-coenzyme A are precursors of acetylcholine. L-Tyrosine, L-dopa and dopamine are precursors of noradrenaline. L-Tryptophan is the precursor of serotonin. L-Tyrosine and L-dopa are precursors of dopamine and histidine is the precursor of histamine.

26. A Biogenic amines

There are three major types of neurotransmitters: biogenic amines, amino acids and peptides. Biogenic amines are well understood and were the first of the neurotransmitters to be discovered.

27. C Hachinski scale

In this scale, there is no requirement for brain imaging.

In the DSM-IV, there must be an evidence of cerebrovascular disease related to dementia aetiologically. According to the ICD-10, features of a dementing illness must be present according to the history, examination and/or tests. Higher cognitive function deficits are unequally distributed, and on clinical examination focal brain damage is found. In the California Criteria, there should be history or clinical evidence of two or more ischaemic strokes. Besides this, at least one infarct outside the cerebellum should be seen on brain imaging. The NINDS/AIREN criteria require evidence of cerebrovascular disease by brain imaging (CT or MRI) or clinical findings of signs of neurological deficits. The findings on brain imaging may include multiple lesions across basal ganglia or large vessel infarcts.

28. B 1972

The CT scan was a great invention in neuroradiology. It came into clinical practice in 1972. It permitted imaging of the brain tissue in live patients. In the present scenario it is the most widely available and widely available imaging tool. A CT scan takes a series of head X-ray from all the vantage points. CT scan are determined by the degree to which any of the tissues absorbs X radiation.

29. E Posterior parietal area

Single photon emission computed tomography findings of reduced regional cerebral blood flow in the posterior parietal and temporal regions help in diagnosis of Alzheimer's disease. The postmortem finding is more reliable in diagnosis than a CT/MRI finding.

30. D γ-Aminobutyric acid concentration is decreased in the caudate nucleus

Huntington's disease is a single gene, autosomal dominant disorder, with complete penetrance (i.e. all carriers of the mutation develop the disease). The mutation is in the gene on chromosome 4p, encoding for a protein called Huntington. This mutation causes a 'trinucleotide repeat' of the codon CAG, which codes for glutamine. Normal individuals have fewer than 30 repeats and disease occurs in individuals having more than 36 copies. Pyramidal neuronal loss occurs in the frontal cortex. There is a reduction in the concentration of the inhibitory transmitter γ-aminobutyric acid in the caudate nucleus. Pyramidal neuronal loss occurs in the frontal cortex. It mainly affects the caudate nucleus and frontal lobes. Caudate nucleus is markedly atrophic and gliotic.

31. E Rate of clonidine metabolism is highest in young children under the age of 6

In adults, 50% of clonidine is metabolised in the liver; 50% is excreted unchanged in the urine. Clonidine has no active metabolites. Its metabolism is highest in young children under the age of 6. As age increases, metabolism decreases. In some children, behavioural withdrawal symptoms due to increased metabolic rates lead to an increase in the frequency of administration of clonidine which is up to four times a day.

32. B They bind to a receptor, and cause an effect in postsynaptic neuron

Neurotransmitters transfer signals across synapses between presynaptic and postsynaptic nerves. By definition, they are synthesised in the presynaptic neuron, stored inactively in the presynaptic nerve ending. When there is a signal and presynaptic nerve ending depolarises, the neurotransmitters are released into the synapse. They bind to a receptor and cause ion channels to open or close and thereby cause transmission of signal. They are degraded in the synapse by enzymes or taken back by presynaptic neuron by reuptake mechanism.

33. E Tyrosine hydroxylase

Hydroxylation of the amino acid L-tyrosine by the enzyme tyrosine hydroxylase leads to production of L-dopa. Dopamine is formed by decarboxylation of L-dopa by dopa decarboxylase. Dopamine β-hydroxylase converts dopamine to noradrenaline in some neurons. Monoamine oxidase or catechol-O-methyl transferase (COMT) inactivates dopamine. Tyrosine hydroxylase is the rate-limiting enzyme in the synthesis of dopamine. Nasrullah et al (1977) tested the dopamine hypothesis of schizophrenia, i.e. there is a functional excess of dopamine. They administered metyrosine (which inhibits tyrosine hydroxylase) to patients with chronic schizophrenia for 3 weeks and found no improvement in schizophrenic symptoms.

34. E Zero-order kinetics

The law of mass action states that the rate of reaction is proportional to the active masses of the reacting substances. This results in zero-order kinetics in which a fixed amount of drug is absorbed or eliminated for each unit of time, independent of the concentration of the drug. Examples include metabolism of alcohol and phenytoin, and absorption of controlled-release drugs and depot antipsychotics. First-order kinetics refers to absorption or elimination of a fixed proportion of drug for each unit of time. Most of the psychiatric medication follow first-order kinetics. Only these two 'order kinetics' are known to date.

35. B Amphetamine

Sensitisation is the enhancement of drug effects following repeated administration of the same dose of drug. Stimulants such as amphetamines cause sensitisation in animals. Tolerance describes a diminished response to the drug after repeated exposure. Repeated use of alcohol, diazepam, heroin and carbamazepine are all associated with development of tolerance. Carbamazepine causes enzyme induction, which leads to increased metabolism with repeated use, and hence dose adjustment is suggested.

36. A Acetazolamide

The excretion of lithium is reduced by all of the above except acetazolamide, which increases the excretion of lithium.

37. E D_2-receptor partial agonist, 5-HT$_{1A}$-receptor agonist, low potential for weight gain, extrapyramidal symptoms and hyperprolactinemia

Bifeprunox is a new antipsychotic, which is a D_2-receptor partial agonist and 5-HT$_{1A}$ agonist. It has minimal propensity to cause weight gain, extrapyramidal symptoms and hyperprolactinemia. Iloperidone is another new antipsychotic and works as D_2-/5-HT$_{2A}$-receptor antagonist with little activity at H$_1$- and muscarinic receptors. It has insomnia as a common adverse effect. Asenapine binds to D_2-, 5-HT$_{2A}$-, 5-HT$_{2C}$- and α_1-/α_2-receptors and has low affinity for H$_1$- and muscarinic receptors. The other two options are distracters.

38. A Cross-taper cautiously

Mirtazapine and venlafaxine can be cross-tapered in either direction. Mirtazapine should be withdrawn and one should wait for a week before starting monoamine oxidase inhibitors (MAOIs). Tricyclic antidepressants (TCAs), reboxetine and selective serotonin reuptake inhibitors (SSRIs) can be started after stopping mirtazapine without wait. While switching to mirtazapine, MAOIs should be withdrawn and mirtazapine can be started after 2 weeks. TCAs, SSRIs (except fluoxetine, 4–7 days wait is recommended), trazodone and reboxetine can be cross-tapered cautiously.

39. E Myocardial infarction

Sildenafil is a phosphodiesterase-5 inhibitor and acts by vasodilatation. It is contraindicated in patients who are on nitrates (can precipitate a sudden fall in blood pressure because both these drugs cause vasodilatation) and patients with a recent history of hypotension, stroke, unstable angina or myocardial infarction. It should be avoided in those patients in whom vasodilatation or sexual activity is inadvisable.

40. C Memantine works by protecting neurons from excessive stimulation

Donepezil, rivastigmine, galantamine and memantine are the drugs used in dementia. They have important differences in their pharmacokinetics and mechanism, which affect their dosing, side effects and indications. Donepezil is highly protein bound whereas rivastigmine circulates mostly unbound. The half-lives of donepezil and rivastigmine are about 70 hours and 1 hour respectively. However, a single dose of rivastigmine will still be effective for 10 hours because it remains bound to cholinesterases. Galantamine acts as an agonist on nicotinic sites and increases the sensitivity of acetylcholine receptors, whereas donepezil and rivastigmine do not. Rivastigmine and galantamine have more peripheral activity outside the central nervous system than donepezil. It explains the favourable adverse effects profile of donepezil, particularly effects on the gastrointestinal tract. Memantine is an N-methyl-D-aspartate antagonist and hence works by protecting neurons from excessive stimulation by glutamate.

41. B Through GABA-B receptors

Carbamazepine acts on GABA-B receptors. This leads to antinociceptive effects. It increases limbic GABA-B receptors, and decreases turnover of dopamine and GABA. It also inhibits inositol transport.

42. E It is a reversible inhibitor of anticholinesterase

Galantamine has dual mode of action. It is a selective reversible inhibitor of acetylcholine esterase. It is also a nicotine acetylcholine receptor agonist, which is responsible for additional benefits in improving cognitive functions.

43. C D_2-receptor partial agonism

Aripiprazole is a D_2-receptor partial agonist. It is a partial agonist at $5HT_{1A}$-receptors and antagonist at $5HT_{2A}$-receptors. It has no anticholinergic effects.

44. D Moclobemide

This is a clinical presentation of hyponatraemia. Most antidepressants have been associated with hyponatraemia; the onset is usually within 30 days of starting treatment. The mechanism of this adverse effect is probably the syndrome of inappropriate secretion of antidiuretic hormone (SIADH). Serotonin is thought to be involved in the regulation of ADH release. Therefore, serotoninergic drugs are relatively more likely to cause this side effect. There are relatively few reports linking MAOIs to hyponatraemia. Old age is a risk factor.

45. B Diarrhoea

Features of serotonin syndrome in order of appearance as the condition worsens are: (1) diarrhoea; (2) restlessness; (3) extreme agitation, hyperreflexia and autonomic instability; (4) myoclonus, seizures, hyperthermia, uncontrollable shivering and rigidity; and (5) delirium, coma, status epilepticus, cardiovascular collapse and death. Concurrent administration of selective serotonin reuptake inhibitors with a monoamine oxidase inhibitor or lithium can precipitate this syndrome.

46. A Coarse tremors

They are suggestive of lithium toxicity whereas fine tremors can be present as side effects at normal therapeutic levels of lithium. All the other effects mentioned in the question are adverse effects of lithium, but may not suggest toxicity. Common indicators of toxicity are vomiting (particularly if it is persistent), abdominal pain, coarse tremors, ataxia, slurred speech, blurred vision, dizziness, nystagmus, convulsions, delirium, circulatory failure and renal failure.

47. E Presynaptic α_2-adrenoreceptor agonism

Clonidine is a presynaptic α_2-receptor agonist. This action is responsible for the sedative action and behavioural effects of clonidine. Clonidine also acts as a postsynaptic α_1-receptor antagonist.

It has high affinity for I_1-type imidazoline receptors. Clonidine's effect on imidazoline receptors contributes to hypotensive effect.

48. C Fluoxetine

Several drugs can cause hyperprolactinaemia. The mechanism includes D_2-receptor blockade, increase in serotonin and potentiation of chemicals such as vasoactive intestinal peptide. Many drugs used in psychiatry cause hyperprolactinaemia and these include antipsychotics, antidepressants such as tricyclics as well as selective serotonin reuptake inhibitors. Opiates and cocaine can cause hyperprolactinaemia. Aripiprazole and haloperidol induce raised prolactin levels. Benzodiazepines decrease the prolactin level due to their GABAergic action, except for alprazolam, which increases prolactin levels. Lithium decreases prolactin levels by an unknown mechanism. Mirtazapine does not cause hyperprolactinaemia and some studies showed that it reduced prolactin.

49. C Olanzapine pamoate

Postinjection delirium/sedation is also known as postinjection syndrome. It can take place after an injection of long-acting olanzapine. It is likely to occur in <0.1% of patients receiving this injection, and does not depend upon the patient's characteristic features. This condition can happen if olanzapine enters the bloodstream too fast. Some of the symptoms seen are: drowsiness, confusion, irritability, restlessness, raised blood pressure and even seizures. Patients are advised to remain at the clinic for 3–5 hours after they have received the injection because symptoms are usually visible by this time if olanzapine has been rapidly absorbed. However, studies have reported that, in 80% of cases, symptoms appear within the first hour of injection. Symptoms tend to resolve and levels of olanzapine return to near normal levels in 1–3 days. The therapeutic action of the long-acting olanzapine injection lasts up to 4 weeks.

50. E Clozapine-related seizures

The side effects mentioned in the options, other than seizures, are not dose related. As the dose of clozapine is increased above 600 mg risk of seizures increases. Clozapine-related seizures are usually managed with sodium valproate.

51. B Neuroleptic malignant syndrome

This is a rare fatal idiosyncratic reaction to a neuroleptic medication. Even though high doses of antipsychotics are a risk factor, neuroleptic malignant syndrome is not dose related. Other side effects, such as extrapyramidal side effects, sedation, postural hypotension, anticholinergic effects, QTc prolongation and sudden cardiac death, are all dose related. Hence one should be very careful when prescribing polypharmacy.

52. D Olanzapine

Of the drugs given above olanzapine is a safer option. Aripiprazole, clozapine and quetiapine are also options to consider when there is history of hyperprolactinaemia with antipsychotic medication.

53. E Topiramate

Aripiprazole prevents manic relapse. Clozapine can be considered in treatment-refractory cases only with due precautions, although there is not a strong evidence base. Lamotrigine is particularly effective in prophylaxis against bipolar depression and bipolar II disorder. Olanzapine is more effective in preventing manic than depressive relapses. Quetiapine can also be used as prophylaxis. Topiramate has been studied as a mood stabiliser but the evidence is not strong enough for a recommendation.

54. D 300 mg

For adult patients taking oral olanzapine 10 mg daily, the initiation would be with 210 mg every 2 weeks or 405 mg every 4 weeks, then a maintenance dose after 2 months' treatment would be 150 mg every 2 weeks or 300 mg every 4 weeks.

For patients taking oral olanzapine 15 mg daily, the initial dose would be 300 mg every 2 weeks and then a maintenance dose after 2 months' treatment could be 210 mg every 2 weeks or 405 mg every 4 weeks.

For patients taking oral olanzapine 20 mg daily, the initial dose would be 300 mg every 2 weeks, then a maintenance dose after 2 months' treatment of 300 mg every 2 weeks. The dose could be adjusted according to the response. The maximum dose is 300 mg every 2 weeks.

Table 4.2 Comparative dosages of oral and depot olanzapine				
Oral	Depot initial dose 2/52	Depot initial dose 4/52	Depot maintenance dose after 2 months 2/52	Depot maintenance dose after 2 months 4/52
10 mg	210	405	150	300
15 mg	300	–	210	405
20 mg	300	–	300	–

55. E Sertraline

The randomised trial for sertraline antidepressant heart attacks is a double-blind randomised control study conducted in patients who had had myocardial infarction (MI) or angina recently. A total of 369 patients with a diagnosis of major depressive disorder were treated with sertraline or placebo for 24 weeks. The study results showed that sertraline was safe and efficacious in patients post-MI or angina. Tricyclics can prolong QTc and cause cardiac arrhythmias.

56. C 30%

A multicentre clinical was conducted by Kane et al (1988) to examine clozapine efficiency in patients with refractory schizophrenia. The study sample in their study was those patients with refractory schizophrenia who had failed to respond to at least three different neuroleptics. These patients initially underwent a prospective, single-blind trial of haloperidol. Patients, who remained unwell even after 6 weeks of haloperidol medication, were then randomly assigned to clozapine or chlorpromazine, in a double-blind manner. Their results showed that 30% of the patients treated with clozapine responded to treatment compared with 4% of patients who received chlorpromazine.

57. D Ecstasy

This is structurally close to amphetamine but has different properties. It causes release of catecholamines (similar to amphetamine) as well as serotonin (similar to hallucinogens). Ecstasy is taken up in serotoninergic neurons by a serotonin transporter responsible for 5HT reuptake and, once inside the neuron, it causes rapid release of a bolus of 5-HT. Cannabis acts on cannabinoid receptors. Cocaine mainly blocks the reuptake of dopamine, but also blocks reuptake of noradrenaline and serotonin. Lysergic acid diethylamide acts as a partial agonist at postsynaptic 5-HT receptors.

58. B It is indicated for the treatment of opioid dependence

It is also indicated for smoking cessation. NICE recommends the use of varenicline for those smokers who wish to quit smoking. It is available as 0.5 mg and 1.0 mg tablets. Varenicline binds at nicotinic acetylcholine receptors, acting as partial agonist. This reduces the symptoms of craving and withdrawal. It is recommended that one course of treatment last for 12 weeks. Its use can cause depression, nausea and vomiting.

59. B Culturing cells in conditions devoid of thymidine

Fragile sites can be present on several chromosomes. One such fragile site is on distal long arm of X chromosome giving rise to the fragile X syndrome. Fragile sites on chromosomes can be demonstrated by culturing cells in conditions of thymidine lack, which can be achieved by using a medium low in thymidine and folic acid, or by adding a thymidine synthetase inhibitor to the culture.

60. D It has two chains of nucleotides wrapped in the form of a double helix, held together by hydrogen bonds

DNA structure consists of two chains of nucleotides bases wrapped in the form of a double helix, held together by hydrogen bonds between the bases. These two chains run in opposite directions. Hydrogen bonds give stability to the helical structure of DNA. There are two classes of nucleobases in DNA. These are purines (adenine and guanine) and pyrimidines (thymine and cytosine). Adenine always pairs with thymine and cytosine with guanine. Base sequence codes genetic information along the DNA molecule.

61. E Deoxyribose sugar, nitrogenous base and a phosphate group

Deoxyribonucleic acid (DNA) consists of a basic repeat unit of deoxyribose sugar, a phosphate group and a nitrogenous base. The nitrogenous base can be adenine, cytosine, guanine or thymine. The order of the nitrogenous bases makes up the DNA sequence.

62. E Ribosomes

Genetic information is expressed by reading it (transcription) and then decoding it (translation). Messenger RNA facilitates the transportation of genetic information from cell nucleus to cytoplasm. Each mRNA molecule is synthesised directly from one strand of DNA, meaning that each mRNA molecule contains a base sequence that is complementary to that particular strand of DNA (gene). This transfer of genetic information from the gene to mRNA is called transcription. Once this mRNA is in the cytoplasm, a protein is synthesised by sequential reading of groups of three bases (a triplet), each coding for a different amino acid with the help of a ribosome, which assembles the different amino acid molecules to form a protein molecule (it may an enzyme or a structural protein), as determined by the respective nucleotide sequence. This is called translation. Some amino acids act as start or stop signals

63. B It is described as diploid

In cell division, the two basic types of cell division are mitosis and meiosis. Mitosis is described as diploid. Daughter cell forms an identical set of chromosomes. Meiosis is described as haploid. Here there is formation of a gamete through parent cell separation.

64. D There is a loss of one base, causing the triplet code to be read out of the frame

Frame-shift mutation is a type of mutation when deletion or addition of nucleotide(s) causes a 'shift' in the reading frame of the triplet codons, resulting in an alteration in the amino acid sequence, thus generating a different protein. A point mutation occurs due to substitution of one base by another. Breaking of a fragment of chromosome and the fragment rejoining at a different site is called translocation. Gaining a piece of DNA is called insertion and loss of a sequence of bases is called deletion.

65. D They can be used to get fragments of easily manageable base-pair sizes (10^3–10^4), thus allowing genes to be handled almost in isolation

Restriction enzymes are also known as restriction endonuclease. It is an enzyme that is found in and used by bacteria to break down infecting viral DNA molecule. Restriction enzymes recognise a specific base sequence and produce a double-stranded cut in the DNA. It cuts double-stranded DNA not at random but rather at specific base sequences sites called restriction sites. A restriction enzyme will recognize a specific base sequence and will cleave at that site. It is of note that it can be used to get fragments of easily manageable base-pair sizes (10^3–10^4), thus allowing genes to be handled almost in isolation.

Around 3000 of these enzymes had been recognized. Many restriction enzymes recognise the same base sequence and thus act at different sites with a similar base sequence; they are known as neoschizomers. There are other restriction enzymes that always recognise and cause cleavage of the DNA segment at the same location every time; these are called isoschizomers. The best use is seen in development of recombinant DNA technology used for producing human insulin by *Escherichia coli* bacteria.

66. B It is used in synthesis of complementary DNA from mRNA

Molecular cloning is a process whereby specific fragments of DNA are biologically purified and amplified, and it usually involves generating bacterial colonies with copies of the specific DNA fragment. Molecular cloning helps in further studies of DNA sequencing of a specific fragment and also as a DNA probe, which is basically a labelled segment of DNA that can be used to find sequence of nucleotides in another specific DNA fragment. There are two main types of DNA probes. First, those derived by using the restriction enzymes and, second, those made from complementary DNA (cDNA), synthesised from mRNA by the action of an enzyme, the 'reverse transcriptase'.

67. C Polymerase chain reaction

Causal mutations are identified by application of molecular genetics. Gross deletions may be detected by Southern blotting, point mutations by DNA sequencing and specific mutations by short oligonucleotide probes. Denaturing gradient gel electrophoresis, chemical cleavage, single-strand conformation analysis and heteroduplex analysis used for identification of causal mutations are based on polymerase chain reaction, which allows us to amplify a single or a few copies of a piece of DNA against a background of a large excess of irrelevant DNA.

68. D It is based on the fact that DNA fragments produced by digestion by a certain restriction enzyme will be of different lengths in different individuals

Restriction fragment length polymorphism (RFLP) analysis is based on the fact that DNA fragments produced by digestion by a certain restriction enzyme will be of different lengths in different individuals. No two individuals' DNA is alike and nor is the length of the DNA fragments. These fragments are detected by Southern blotting. RFLPs are generally inherited in a mendelian fashion so they can be used as genetic markers. It is a kind of DNA fingerprinting and is used to identify whether a sample of DNA came from a particular individual. Most RFLPs arise due to single base substitutions. Positional cloning is a technique that identifies disease genes by their position on a genome rather than through their function

69. D Mutation of a gene

Imprinting is the process by which genes are made inactive and this is reversible. Imprinted genes are not expressed. It does not affect the sequence of DNA, and takes place during gametogenesis. Imprinting is an epigenetic principle and inactivation is by methylation and histone modification.

70. B Candidate gene association studies

In allelic association, a sample of individuals affected by a disorder (cases) is compared with controls who do not have the disorder. The most useful test is measuring relative risk or the odds ratio. The commonest type of association study in psychiatry is the candidate gene association approach. Whole genome association studies are basically a systematic search to determine linkage disequilibrium or direct association. Population stratification is the presence of a systematic difference in allele frequencies between cases and controls due to ancestry difference, and is usually due to non-random mating between groups. Multiple testing can be applied when many single nucleotide polymorphisms are considered at once and they might be exhibiting linkage disequilibrium. If the multiple testing is not adjusted appropriately, it may produce excessive false positives or false negatives.

71. C 40%

In a meta-analysis by Rhee and Waldman, the heritability for antisocial behaviours was found to be 0.41 and the environmental contribution was 0.59. Antisocial personality disorder and antisocial behaviours are mainly found in young men. Social factors determine the degree of expression for antisocial behaviour in women. Torgersen et al (2000) showed the heritability of borderline personality disorder to be of the order of 0.69 which rose to 0.80 on using strict criteria for diagnosis.

72. A Antisocial behaviour

To date the strongest evidence for a gene and environment interaction for a gene variant that affects monoamine oxidase A gene enzymatic activity comes from the increased risk of antisocial behaviour only in the presence of childhood maltreatment. A gene variant has also been found that affects the serotonin transporter, increasing the risk of depression at times of life events. Adults who have a genotype conferring a low MAOA activity and also suffered childhood abuse have a high risk for aggression and antisocial behaviour. At the other end of the scale, a person who was abused as a child but has high levels of MAOA activity will be less likely to develop antisocial behaviour.

73. B Hunter's syndrome

This is a lysosomal storage disease and has X-linked inheritance; it is due to a deficiency of iduronate-2-sulphatase. Compared with Hurler's disease, there is slower progression of symptoms and less occurrence of learning disability. Symptoms are very similar to Hurler's syndrome and the urine contains heparin and dermatan sulphate. Hunter's syndrome is always severe, progressive, and life limiting. All the other metabolic diseases are autosomal recessive.

74. E Two or more mutant alleles exist at the same locus, resulting in different phenotypes

Genetic heterogeneity is a big problem in linkage studies. When two or more mutant alleles exist at the same locusm resulting in different phenotypes, it is called allelic heterogeneity, e.g. less severe Becker muscular dystrophy and Duchene muscular dystrophy both occur due to a mutation in the X chromosome and at the same locus. When allelic mutation at two or more loci results in a similar phenotype, it is called locus heterogeneity, e.g. tuberous sclerosis and retinitis pigmentosa, both of which can result from different mutations on different chromosomes. Some disorders, however, might have a major locus but most of cases are either polygenic or not genetic at all, e.g. breast carcinoma and Alzheimer's disease.

75. C The phenomenon that affected individuals is found in every generation

In autosomal dominant disorders, every generation will have some individuals affected by the disorder. This is called vertical transmission.

76. B Expressivity

In people who manifest with clinical phenotypes, different individuals may present with varying degrees of symptom manifestation, i.e. from mild to severe form, having few symptoms to many symptoms. This is called expressivity. A good example is that of neurofibromatosis.

77. B RNA polymerase II

Three main steps in transcription of RNAs are initiation, mRNA chain elongation and termination. Three different RNA polymerases, I, II and III, carry out transcription. All these three polymerases serve different functions. Large ribosomal RNAs are encoded by genes with the help of polymerase I. Protein synthesis is done with the help of polymerase II. Other RNAs such as snRNAs, tRNAs and small rRNAs are encoded with the help of polymerase III.

78. E There is mating among professionals with a high IQ

The Hardy–Weinberg equilibrium is disturbed when there is mutation, natural selection and non-random mating. Gene flow and genetic drift can also disturb the equilibrium. Gene frequencies can be altered due to natural selection or non-random mating, and hence disrupt the equilibrium. The Hardy–Weinberg equilibrium rarely applies in reality simply because all factors mentioned above are commonly present in nature. The equilibrium therefore describes an idealised state. In the above question, mating among professionals with a high IQ will lead to fewer and fewer allelic frequencies of average or low IQs, hence disrupting the equilibrium.

79. D Prepulse inhibition

Usually when a sudden and unexpected noise or light stimulates a person, startle response occurs. This response can be blunted or inhibited by exposing the person to a weaker stimulus 100 ms before the stronger stimulus. In patients with schizophrenia and their families, this diminution is attenuated. Other terms mentioned are actual psychopathological terms

80. E Sortilin-related receptor (*SORL1*) gene

This is also known as SORLA and LR11. It is involved in movement of amyloid precursor protein in the cells. In the event of suppression of the *SORL1* gene, there is an increased production of toxic amyloid β precursor. This in turn has been associated with an increased risk of Alzheimer's dementia.

81. B 14%

Gottesman reviewed the literature and calculated the average probandwise concordance rate of schizophrenia. It is 46% in monozygotic twins and 14% in dizygotic twins.

82. D Epigenetics

This is a study of epigenesis. In today's world epigenetics encapsulates studying any changes in DNA or associated proteins. These changes are inheritable. Epigenetic mechanisms at the molecular level can be methylation, modification of histones and non-coding. From a research point of view, epigenetic effects of cannabis can be identified by either post-mortem brain cells or live cells such as buccal mucosa cells.

83. B 1%

The single most predictive factor for the development of schizophrenia is family history of schizophrenia. However, patients with 22Q deletion syndrome have no family history of schizophrenia. They form 1% of the population of patients with schizophrenia.

84. B 50%

Huntington's disease is an autosomal dominant disorder. For autosomal dominant disorders to manifest only one disease, an allele is necessary. In most instances, when one affected parent is a heterozygote for the disease, and the other parent does not have the illness, approximately 50% of the children show the disorder.

85. E Analysis of the gene–environment interaction using statistical techniques

Path analysis is a statistical technique used in genetics to estimate the size of genetic and environmental components in causing mental disorders, i.e. the effect of gene and environment variation. It is shown using a path diagram. This is similar to regression analysis, used in statistics.

86. B Centimorgans

Genetic distances are measured using the unit known as centimorgans; 1 centimorgan is equivalent to recombination occurring in every 100 meiotic divisions, i.e. recombination fraction of 0.01.

87. B It is defined as the number of recombinants divided by the total number of offspring

During meiotic division, there is crossing over of genetic material. The offspring who have the new combination of genetic material are called recombinants. Offspring with genetic material the same as the parents are called non-recombinants. The recombination fraction is simply defined as the number of recombinants divided by the total number of offspring.

88. A −2

Logarithm of odds (LOD) score was described by Newton E Mortonin in 1955. The LOD score is a statistical test that helps to calculate linkage distances. It is a technique used in human, plant and animal linkage studies. The presence of linkage is suggested by a +LOD score whereas the chances of linkage are likely to be less if −LOD scores are found.

89. C 0.5

Genotypic correlation between dizygotic twins as well as siblings is 0.5, i.e. they have 50% genes in common. Genotypic correlation for monozygotic twins is 1. They have 100% genes common to both.

90. E Liability to develop schizophrenia that presents from childhood

Originally Paul Meehl used the word schizotaxia to describe the liability to develop schizophrenia or a schizophrenia-like conditions. Gene–environment interactions lead to development of schizophrenia or schizophrenia-like disorders in susceptible individuals. This susceptibility is expressed through a combination of cognitive, neurobiological and social skills deficits in childhood and this is called schizotaxia.

91. D Qualitative study

Qualitative research is also known as interpretive research. It tries to study things in their natural setting, attempting to make sense of, or interpret, phenomena in terms of the meanings that people bring to them. The data are usually gathered with semi-structured individual interviews, in focus group sessions or by simple observations. Such observations may not be generalised to wider populations, but may generate a hypothesis for further testing.

92. C It varies systematically with exposure and acts as an independent risk or protective factor for the disease

A confounder is a variable that is associated with both exposure and outcome, but not on the causal pathway. Restricting the study population sample can reduce the influence of the confounders. Age and sex are the common confounders.

93. D Mixed anxiety and depressive disorder

The frequency of neurotic condition in descending order is mixed anxiety and depression 48%, GAD 28%, depression14%, phobias 12%, OCD 10% and panic disorder 6%.

94. C Prisoners and homeless

The incidence of developing neurotic illness increases with increasing environmental stress. All the above factors are associated with the development of neurotic disorder. The risk is twice for prisoners and homeless.

95. C 10%

About 10% of the general population have specific phobias. The lifetime prevalence is 11.3%. The 12-month national co-morbidity survey (NCS) prevalence is 8.8% and the 6-month epidemiological catchment area study (ECA) prevalence is 4.5–11.9%. In the DSM- IV, there are five types of specific phobias mentioned:

1. animals
2. aspects of the natural environment
3. blood, injection and injury
4. situations
5. other provoking agents.

Animal and social phobias are more common in females.

96. B Cause-specific mortality rate

This refers to the ratio of the number of deaths due to a particular disease, e.g. depression, in a given population and those in the total population. The crude mortality rate is the ratio of deaths due to all causes in a given population and those in the total population. The case fatality rate refers to comparison of the number of deaths in patients with a given diagnosis with the total number of patients with the same diagnosis. The proportional mortality rate refers to the comparison of number of deaths in patients with a condition with deaths due to all causes in the population.

97. A Electroencephalography abnormalities are less common in vCJD

Variant Creutzfeldt–Jakob disease (vCJD) has an earlier onset. It has a slower course. The 'pulvinar sign' on MRI is a useful diagnostic sign in vCJD. The vCJD usually presents with psychiatric symptoms including depression and personality changes. Bovine spongiform encephalopathy (BSE) and vCJD are caused by the same prion strain and there is no doubt that vCJD occurs on eating contaminated beef products. Usually there is a polymorphism at codon 129 of the prion protein (PrP) gene encoding for either methionine or valine, whereas almost all patients with vCJD are homozygous at codon 129 of the PrP gene that encodes for methionine. Electroencephalography abnormalities are less common in vCJD.

98. C 50–70%

Transvestism is sometimes seen among obsessive personalities. Some studies suggest that around 50–70% of transvestites can be diagnosed as having a personality disorder.

99. A Mid-20s

It has been suggested that about 50% of all mental illness arises by the age of 14 years and about 75% of all lifetime illnesses by the mid-20s. When measured in 2004, nearly a quarter of the burden of disease in the UK was due to mental health disorder, and this was higher than cardiovascular diseases or cancer.

100. D 20

Studies have shown that suicide is a major public health issue and a significant cause of death. Rates of suicide and self-harm are higher in certain age groups compared with others. When compared with a normal population, people with severe mental health disorders have a 20-fold higher rate of suicide. The rate is even higher (30-fold) in those who have history of self-harm. In prisoners the rates of suicide are higher in women (20 times) compared with men (5 times). Other groups that are at a higher risk of suicide are young men and those from black and ethnic minority groups. There has been a significant rise in self-harm by young people in the last decade.

101. C 50%

Smoking is a preventable illness. On an average the lifespan of a smoker is 10 years less than that of a non-smoker. The prevalence of smoking in the general population is 21%. The prevalence of smoking is highest in those who have a mental illness and are in prison (80%), or attend methadone maintenance clinics (80%). The rate of smoking is around 70% in those who are inpatients on mental health wards. Roughly half of all tobacco consumed in the UK is by those who have mental illness.

102. E Road traffic accidents are the commonest cause of head injury

Around 200–300/100,000 people attend hospitals every year for head injury. About one-sixth of them will need admission. About 80% of head injuries are mild, 10% moderate and 10% severe. Road traffic accidents are by far the largest cause of head injuries, followed by assaults and falls. A significant number of people also get head injury due to deliberate self-harm. Alcohol misuse and lower socioeconomic status are high risk factors. Around 100/100,000 people have considerable disability due to head injury.

103. B Risk is higher for first-generation migrants than for second-generation migrants

Relative risk for first-generation migrants is 2.7 compared with 4.5 in the second-generation migrants. Risk is higher for migrants from a lower socioeconomic status and in black people moving to dominantly white countries. Also, there is a greater risk in siblings rather than the parents of the second generation.

104. C Ecological fallacy

Central limit theorem indicates that, as a sample size increases, the mean approaches a normal distribution. According to the theorem, this is independent of the shape of the distribution. A ceiling effect is an undesirable measurement outcome, occurring when the people on a measurement have reached the maximum possible value. For example, a memory test that assesses how many words a participant can recall has a total of five words that each participant is asked to remember. As most individuals can remember all five words, this measure has a ceiling effect.

105. C 1100/89,000

The incidence rate of the disease is the number of people who develop an illness in a given time period divided by the total number of individuals at risk for the illness during that time period. In the above question, there were 90,000 people in a town. In 2009, there were 1000 people who were diagnosed with melanoma. In 2010, 89,000 people were at risk of developing this condition. The incidence rate in 2010 would be 1100/89,000.

106. E 2100/90,000

The prevalence rate is calculated by adding the diagnoses of patient in 2009 (1000) and 2010 (1100) divided by the total population at risk. The prevalence rate in 2010 would be (1000 + 1100)/90,000.

107. B 4

The relative risk compares the incidence rate of a disorder among individuals exposed to risk factors, with the incidence rate of the disorder in those who are not exposed. In this example, the chance of developing schizophrenia (relative risk) for the population would be 80/1000 divided by 20/1000 which will be 4. It means that if a person smokes cannabis he is four times at risk of developing schizophrenia than another person who does not use cannabis.

108. C 60

The attribution risk helps to determine what would happen in a given population if the risk factor were removed. The attribution risk is calculated by subtracting the incidence rate of people who are exposed to the risk factors (80/1000) from the incidence of those who are not exposed (20/1000). The attribution risk would be 60/1000.

109. C 41–50

Global assessment of functioning scale is used to measure social, occupational and psychological functioning. The values on the scale range from 0 to 100. The higher the value the better the person's functioning. For example, 0–10 would mean persistent risk to self or others; 21–30 would suggest serious impairment in judgement and almost no ability in functioning; 41–50 suggests serious impairment in functioning in various areas or the person has serious symptoms. The scale can also be used to measure clinical progress in individuals. It is supposed to measure the level of functioning at the time of assessment, i.e. current period.

110. D Wada test

The Halstead–Reitan neuropsychological battery is used to assess the location of a brain lesion and its effects by 10 tests that measure various neurological functions. It may also help to differentiate depression and early dementia. The Wada test by Juhn Wada (1924) confirms the cerebral dominance in an individual patient, helping to decide on destructive brain surgery. After infusion of amobarbital into the carotid artery of the dominant side, there is step-wise transient aphasia in seconds to minutes. The word association test was developed by Carl Jung; in this the person is given a stimulus word and requested to respond with the 'first' word that comes to his or her mind. Electrophysiological testing is a study of abnormal patterns on standard EEG, which measures and characterises cognitive decline.

111. D Publication bias

A funnel plot works on the assumption that, if all studies conducted about a similar subject were represented graphically by plotting respective effect magnitude against respective sample size, a funnel-shaped distribution would be formed. Publication bias is particularly relevant to systematic reviews. It occurs because studies reporting positive findings are more likely to be accepted for publication in journals than studies that report negative findings.

112. C Kaplan–Meier curve

Survival probabilities are calculated only when the event of interest occurs in a study. Survival probabilities just before the event are brought forward and adjusted using the post-event survival rate of the remaining uncensored participants. It is this repeated carrying over of survival probabilities that creates a cumulative value, which can be represented pictorially as a Kaplan–Meier survival curve.

113. D Neuroticism

Based on Eysenk's three personality traits, the five big personality factors can be identified over time. Eysenk's three traits are extraversion, neuroticism and psychoticism. The table below provides details of the five big personality traits.

Table 4.4 Eysenck's personality traits and big personality factors

Factor	Desirable trait	Undesirable trait
Neuroticism (or emotional stability)	Calm, even tempered	Anxious, moody, impulsive, temperamental
Extraversion	Outgoing, social, assertive	Introverted, reserved, passive
Openness to experience	Imaginative, intelligent, creative	Shallow, unsophisticated, unperceptive
Agreeableness	Kind, trusting, warm, altruistic	Hostile, selfish, cold
Conscientiousness	Organised, thorough, tidy, competent	Careless, unreliable, sloppy

114. A Anxiety disorders

A pilot study was conducted by Comtois et al (2003) to identify factors associated with high rates of inpatient admission in people with borderline personality disorders. The sample size was 29 and included both Spanish- and English-speaking people. More than half of the sample had high rates of inpatient admission. The results revealed that high levels of admission to wards were associated with a history of parasuicide in the preceding 2 years, the presence of anxiety disorders and poorer cognitive functioning. The high rates were not associated with severity of para suicides, depressive symptoms and psychosis, or substance misuse problems.

115. C Specialist partial treatment for borderline personality disorder is no more expensive than treatment as usual and shows considerable cost savings after treatment

Bateman and Fonagy (2003) compared the health care utilisation of patients with borderline personality disorder in a partial hospital treatment setting with treatment as usual. They found that there was no difference in pre- and post-treatment in the two groups. The increased cost of partial hospitalisation was offset by reduced psychiatric inpatient admissions and emergency care. The authors concluded that specialist partial hospital treatment for borderline personality disorder is similar in cost to treatment as usual. Furthermore, it showed a cost saving after the treatment.

116. C Antipsychotic drug

Symptoms of schizotypal personality disorder such as ideas of reference and illusions can be treated with antipsychotic medication. Koenigsberg et al (2003) conducted a randomised controlled study that showed significant benefit of risperidone in patients with schizotypal personality disorder. An antipsychotic can be used together with psychotherapy for treatment of schizotypal disorder. In the presence of comorbid depression, an antidepressant may be beneficial.

117. E Mentalisation-based therapy (MBT) with partial hospitalisation is effective in reducing suicide attempts and self-harm

There is a relatively poor evidence base for psychological therapies for treating borderline personality disorders. Some studies have shown that therapies such as dialectical behavioural therapy (DBT) and MBT with partial hospitalisation reduce suicide attempts, self-harm, anger, aggression and depressive symptoms. It has been suggested that DBT is effective in reducing self-harm and should be considered for women in whom self-harm is a major problem.

118. E Self-esteem: social acceptance

According to Maslow, there is a hierarchy of needs. The lower-order needs must be satisfied before it is possible to satisfy higher-order needs.

Table 4.5 Maslow's hierarchy of needs in descending order

Order	Example
1. Self-actualisation	Achievement
2. Aesthetic	Symmetry, order
3. Cognitive	Knowledge, understanding
4. Self-esteem	Social acceptance, recognition
5. Belonging/social	Group membership, affiliation
6. Safety	Security, absence of danger
7. Physical/physiological	Hunger, thirst

119. B Authoritative

The authoritative parental style tends to result in children being happier, more capable and successful. The authoritative style involves rules and boundaries that are executed in a more democratic way. Parents are willing to listen to their children and are more responsive. With the authoritarian style, parents are stricter about following rules, without an explanation as to why these rules need to be followed. They have high demands and are not responsive to their children. The children, in this case, tend to be obedient and proficient, but are less happy with low self-esteem. Indulgent and neglectful are also parental styles.

120. B Child can develop depression in later life

Children of postnatally depressed mothers show less behavioural disturbances than those with mothers whose illness evolved via different pathways.

Children whose mothers are concurrently depressed show:

- poorer cognitive outcomes
- more behavioural disturbances
- more insecure attachments
- more difficult temperaments
- greater risk of developing depression later in life.

121. C If identified and treated early, puerperal psychosis is relatively benign

Puerperal psychosis is the acute onset of psychotic symptoms after childbirth. If not identified and treated, psychotic symptoms can continue for several months with significant deterioration in functioning. However, it can resolve within a few days if adequately treated. Bipolar illness, similar to manic illness, has benign effects on the mother's relationship with the infant. Postnatal depressive illness can have delayed effects and may contribute to late-onset behavioural problems in the infant.

122. D Postnatal depression is more apparent in children coming from deprived backgrounds

The following are known agents in the explanatory model of how a mother influences the development of child psychopathology:

- Maternal mental illness directly provokes child psychopathology, e.g. infanticide in postnatal depression
- Maternal mental illness indirectly impairs children via disturbed attachments
- Maternal mental illness causes general parenting impediments and therefore in turn impairs attachments
- Maternal mental illness distorts child development, e.g.poor cognitive development in children whose mothers were postnatally depressed
- Common genetic loading expressed differently at different ages
- Mentally ill mothers are less effective at protecting their children from adversity.

123. E Ill or disabled children

The following are known agents in the explanatory model of how a child influences the development of psychopathology in the mother:

- Childbirth as an insult
- Difficult child temperament in abuse and maternal mental illness
- Parenting problems and humiliation from child behaviour contributing to maternal mental

illness
- Impact of children on marital intimacy
- Ill or disabled children.

124. A Ainsworth

The strange situation test and adult attachment interview were described by Ainsworth. The strange situation test explores the concepts of attachment proposed by Bowlby. Harlow, through his experiments in monkeys, showed that infants need both warmth and food. Rutter studied the effects of maternal privation and deprivation on children.

125. E There are reciprocal relationships between a baby and the environment

Thomas and Chess described the goodness of fit when a reciprocal relationship between a child and its environment, especially with the mother, exists. This is different to the concept of the good-enough mother proposed by Winnicott.

The EAS model (**Figure 4.1**) describes the three-dimensions of temperament such as emotionality, activity and sociability.

A difficult temperament in a child may adapt to a harsh environment and help with survival.

126. B Inner working models of attachment

According to Bowlby, inner working models are formed from our early experiences of caregiving, which are carried forward onto new relationships during our lifetime. These working models then affect our perception and behaviour. Bem, a behavioural therapist, devised the self-perception theory. Sigmund Freud devised the theory of motivation. Hobbes devised the theory of hedonism. Tolman described cognitive behaviourism and social learning.

127. E Shadow

Carl Jung described the unconscious impulses towards a psychic counterpart called an archetype, such as shadow, the self, the anima, the animus and the persona. Melanie Klein was particularly concerned with describing the earliest infantile conflicts and anxieties. Klein's contributions to psychoanalysis include the concept of internal object and the internal world, the primitive mental processes of splitting and projective identification, and the paranoid–schizoid and depressive position.

128. A Attachment and effects of early experiences

Freud is known for his contribution with theories on motivation, dreams and the relationship between sleep and dreams, attachment and effects of early experiences, moral and gender development, and aggression. Stephen Jay Gould is known for his theory on evolution of adult consciousness. According to Gould, adult consciousness evolves as the person releases him- or herself from the constraints and ties of childhood consciousness.

129. D Gambling is an example of variable-ratio reinforcement

Resistance to extinction is very high in variable-interval and variable-ratio reinforcement. In this case, the response is reinforced after an unpredictable number of responses. In continuous reinforcement, resistance to extinction is very low, and every single response is reinforced. Being regularly paid is a type of fixed interval reinforcement, which has a low resistance to extinction. Piecework and commissioning are examples of fixed-ratio reinforcement.

130. C Displacement

In dreams, the underlying (latent) wishes are converted to manifest content. Displacement happens in dreams in which the real target is substituted by a person or an object that becomes the target of those feelings. In condensation, more than one dream may be 'condensed' into a single manifest image. Concrete representation refers to expression of an abstract idea in a concrete way.

131. A Clinic privileges

Contingency management in patients with drug misuse uses four methods of providing incentives if a patient remains abstinent from the illicit drug. One of the methods is clinic incentive which includes direct benefits from the clinic such as taking methadone home on providing a negative sample. Another method is a voucher-based incentive in which patients receive vouchers with a monetary value. Prize-based incentive includes lottery-style tickets, which have a 50% chance of winning some money. Finally, the patients may also receive direct monies as part of the incentive.

132. A Contingency management is associated with continuous periods of abstinence in cocaine misuse

When considering psychological therapies for patients with drug misuse, behavioural couples therapy can be considered where the partner is supportive and willing to participate in the therapy. Social systems intervention includes people who are involved in the care of young people such as parents, carers, teachers or friends. Neither relapse-prevention nor standard cognitive behavioural therapy has been found to be effective for the treatment of cocaine dependence. Various studies have shown that, for cocaine misusers, contingency management has been shown to be effective.

133. E There is limited evidence that individual supportive psychotherapy is superior to family therapy in terms of weight gain

Psychological therapy in patients with anorexia nervosa is aimed at not only weight gain and healthy eating, but also promoting psychological health. Few studies have compared family interventions and focal psychoanalytic psychotherapy with treatment as usual and have found them effective. There is insufficient evidence in adult populations with regard to any one effective therapy. However, research on weight gain points towards supportive psychological therapy being better than family therapy.

134. C Focal psychodynamic psychotherapy

An effective therapy suggested for patients with anorexia nervosa (AN) is focal psychodynamic psychotherapy. It is a time-limited psychodynamic psychotherapy. Other therapies that have shown benefit in AN patients include cognitive–analytic therapy, cognitive–behavioural therapy (CBT) and interpersonal therapy. For bulimia nervosa, psychological therapies considered include CBT–bulimia nervosa (CBT–BN), CBT with exposure and response prevention, guided self-help and simplified dialectical behaviour therapy.

135. B CBT-BN is superior to dietary counselling for managing purging by the end of the treatment

There is strong evidence that CBT–BN is superior to interpersonal therapybulimia nervosa (IPT-BN) in terms of remission from binge eating and purging. CBT–BN is superior to dietary counselling for managing purging by the end of treatment but not by the end of follow-up. CBT–BN is no more acceptable than other forms of psychotherapy or dietary counselling.

136. B Sixteen to twenty sessions of both psychodynamic psychotherapy and CBT are insufficient for most patients to achieve lasting remission

No significant difference has been found in a meta-analytic study between short-term psychodynamic psychotherapy and CBT on effects of depressive symptoms and social functioning, and in terms of patient remission or improvement. Sixteen to twenty sessions of both therapies were found to be insufficient for most patients to achieve lasting remission.

137. B For more complex interventions, therapists require longer training to be competent therapists

Therapist training is more important than personal attributes and styles. Some complex therapies require therapists who have trained for longer periods than others. These therapies include trauma-focused CBT and CBT for psychotic illnesses. CBT research has focused on its development rather than its mechanism of action. Studies that have compared styles of CBTs have shown that self-study CBT can be as good as full CBT if given along with a few individual sessions. However, for post-traumatic stress disorder, a skilled therapist is needed for a good outcome.

138. A Sixteen to twenty sessions of psychotherapy are required for optimal effects of psychotherapy

In a recent meta-analysis, psychotherapy has been found to be less effective than pharmacotherapy, especially selective serotonin reuptake inhibitors, for patients with depression and dysthymia. Combined treatment is better than pharmacotherapy and even more so than psychotherapy. About 18 sessions of psychotherapy are required to see optimal effects of psychotherapy in patients with depression.

139. C It is an emotional experience that establishes the nature of a relationship between phenomena or objects

Bion introduced the term 'linking'. It is specifically employed to discuss the patient's relationship with functions such as endurance, fortitude, patience, danger, love and empathy. Love (L), hate (H) and knowledge (K) are the three links that represent the dynamic relationship between psychoanalytical objects and container.

140. C CBT

A recent randomised control trial compared CBT, behavioural weight loss and a combination of both. The study involved a 12-month follow-up of 15 patients who were randomly assigned to the three groups. The results revealed that CBT was better at reducing binge eating than behavioural weight loss (BWL). However, the BWL method was superior to CBT alone in reducing weight in patients during the trial. It was noted that 51% of the patients with binge eating who were treated with CBT achieved remission. The remission rates were 36–40% for those who had BWL and a sequential CBT and BWL.

141. C CBT was found to be neither inferior nor superior to applied relaxation

On comparison with CBT applied relaxation therapy had similar outcomes in patients with generalised anxiety disorder. Studies have shown that CBT is effective in patients with generalised anxiety disorder compared with waiting. For short-term outcomes, CBT has also been found to be more effective at reducing anxiety and depressive features than psychodynamic psychotherapy.

Chapter 5

Mock examination

Questions: MCQs

For each question, select one answer option.

1. Which of the following chromosomal disorders is due to trisomy 21?

   A   Down's syndrome
   B   Edwards' syndrome
   C   Meta-female
   D   Patau's syndrome
   E   Turner's syndrome

2. In which of the following conditions is interpersonal therapy an effective treatment?

   A   Childhood sexual abuse
   B   Death of a loved one
   C   Encopresis
   D   Misuse of illicit drugs
   E   Short-term memory problems

3. An 18-year-old male college student presented with depressed mood, tiredness, paranoid delusions, abnormal movements, clumsiness and rigidity. He did not have any past psychiatric history. Which of the following is most appropriate treatment?

   A   Benzatropine
   B   Penicillamine
   C   Prednisolone
   D   Quetiapine
   E   Tetrabenazine

4. Which of the following is licensed for the treatment of tardive dyskinesia in UK?

   A   Benzodiazepines
   B   Botulinum toxin
   C   Pyridoxine
   D   Tetrabenazine
   E   Vitamin E

5. Blockage of which of the following arteries results in the lateral medullary syndrome?

   A   Anteroinferior cerebral artery
   B   Anterior cerebral artery
   C   Middle cerebral artery
   D   Posterior cerebral artery
   E   Posteroinferior cerebellar artery

6. Which of the following statements about the WAGR syndrome is correct?

    A   Deletion on short arm of chromosome 15 when a child presents with craniofacial abnormalities, microcephaly, learning disability and abnormal cry
    B   Deletion on the long arm of paternal chromosome 11 when a child presents with reduced height, smaller hands, feet and testicles, infantile hypotonia and angry outbursts
    C   There is deletion on chromosome 11 which can lead to bilateral retinoblastoma with reduced IQ
    D   There is deletion of chromosome 11, and it presents with aniridia, reduced IQ and ambiguous genitalia
    E   There is deletion of the long arm of chromosome 11 with hypertelorism, ptosis macrocephaly and epicanthal folds

7. Which of the following therapies was developed by Moreno?

    A   Couple's therapy
    B   Group therapy
    C   Play therapy
    D   Psychodrama
    E   Reminiscence therapy

8. What is the most sensitive and specific diagnostic procedure for variant Creutzfeldt-Jakob disease?

    A   Electroencephalography
    B   Hepatic biopsy
    C   Human PrP gene (*PRNP*) analysis
    D   MRI of the brain
    E   Tonsillar biopsy

9. Friedreich's ataxia is linked to the abnormality of an identified gene. Which of the following is the abnormal gene?

    A   Ataxin 1
    B   *DMPIL*
    C   *FMRP*
    D   Frataxin
    E   Huntingtin

10. Which of the following refers to transference?

    A   Affective resonance and empathy
    B   Emergence of latent meanings
    C   Part of the bipersonal or intersubjective field
    D   The results of projective identification
    E   The analyst's blind spot or resistance

11. Which of the following antipsychotic drugs is synthesised from pethidine?

    A   Chlorpromazine
    B   Haloperidol
    C   Risperidone
    D   Thioridazine
    E   Trifluoperazine

12. Which is the largest nuclear mass in the central nervous system?

    A   Brain stem
    B   Cerebral cortex

    C   Cerebellum
    D   Hypothalamus
    E   Thalamus

13. Who proposed the dual representation theory of post-traumatic stress disorder?

    A   Brewin
    B   Capgras
    C   Folstein
    D   Roth
    E   Williams

14. What is the neurobiological substrate of memory impairment in depression?

    A   Cerebellar atrophy
    B   Frontal lobe deviation
    C   Left hippocampal density
    D   Medial cerebral artery thickening
    E   Temporal lobe enlargement

15. Which of the following is a mature ego defence mechanism according to Vaillant's hierarchy of defences?

    A   Displacement
    B   Projection
    C   Reaction formation
    D   Repression
    E   Suppression

16. Which of the following statements about behavioural phenotypes is correct?

    A   Gaze aversion is a very noticeable feature of fragile X syndrome
    B   Hand and hand to mouth stereotypies occur in phenylketonuria
    C   Hyperphagia and compulsive behaviour occur in Angelman's syndrome
    D   Self-mutilation of fingers and lips occurs in Williams' syndrome
    E   Superficial sociability, hyperlalia and language disorder occur in Down's syndrome

17. What is the process whereby an analyst's feelings are aroused when a patient projects his or her feelings onto the therapist?

    A   Countertransference
    B   Dissociation
    C   Dream interpretation
    D   Resistance
    E   Therapeutic alliance

18. Which of the following is not involved in the genetic transmission of schizophrenia?

    A   Catecholamine hydroxylase gene
    B   Catecholamine-O-methyl transferase
    C   Dysbindin ($DTNBP1$)
    D   G72 (D-amino acid oxidase activator)
    E   Neuregulin (NRG1)

19. An 11-year-old boy was brought to child psychiatry services by his parents with well-defined symptoms of schizophrenia. Which of the following antipsychotics is licenced for use in this age group?

    A   Aripiprazole

    B   Haloperidol
    C   Olanzapine
    D   Quetiapine
    E   Risperidone

20. Which of the following features indicates the use of supportive psychotherapy in preference to analytic psychotherapy?

    A   Good impulse control
    B   Good psychological mindedness
    C   Intact reality testing
    D   Meaningful object relations
    E   Poor frustration tolerance

21. Which of the following results from damage to the arcuate fasciculus?

    A   Conduction dysphasia
    B   Expressive dysphasia
    C   Global dysphasia
    D   Nominal dysphasia
    E   Receptive dysphasia

22. In which of the following drug uses does a patient experience flashbacks?

    A   Amphetamine
    B   Cannabis
    C   Cocaine
    D   Ecstasy
    E   Heroine

23. What type of clinical trials are CATIE and CUtLASS studies?

    A   Phase 1 clinical trial
    B   Phase 2 clinical trial
    C   Phase 3 clinical trial
    D   Phase 4 clinical trial
    E   Preclinical trial

24. Which of the following is a characteristic feature of Maslow's self-actualisers?

    A   Accept themselves and others for what they are
    B   Deep appreciation of the materialistic experiences of life
    C   Do not enjoy solitude
    D   Enjoy company of others for self-development
    E   Unpredictable in thought and behaviour

25. Who described the concept of containment?

    A   Anna Freud
    B   Bion
    C   Daniel stern
    D   Jung
    E   Melanie Klein

26. A 24-year-old man always had an extreme fear of dogs. Which of the following is a term used for this condition?

    A   Arachnophobia
    B   Cyanophobia

    C   Herpetophobia
    D   Ophidiophobia
    E   Zemmiphobia

27. Which of the following circuits is related to the amygdala?

    A   Cognitive loop
    B   Emotional circuit
    C   Limbic loop
    D   Motor loop
    E   Oculomotor loop

28. Which of the following statements about genes is correct?

    A   A recessive gene is expressed even if it is present on only one chromosome
    B   Genes encode for multiple sets of proteins
    C   They form 10% of total human DNA
    D   They have DNA segments that do not code for amino acids–called exons
    E   They have DNA segments that do not code for amino acids–called introns

29. Which of the following is the right order for the three Rs of cognitive analytical therapy?

    A   Recognition, reformulation and revision
    B   Recognition, revision and reformulation
    C   Reformulation, recognition and revision
    D   Reformulation, revision and recognition
    E   Revision, recognition and reformulation

30. Which of the following is included in the gestalt awareness cycle?

    A   Content
    B   Movement
    C   Recognition
    D   Retreat
    E   Sensation

31. Which of the following is a characteristic feature of upper motor neuron lesions?

    A   Absence of clumsiness
    B   Clonus
    C   Cremasteric reflexes
    D   Fasciculation
    E   Abdominal reflexes

32. A 27-year-old man presented with schizophrenia. He was treated with haloperidol, quetiapine and amisulpride in therapeutic doses on separate occasions. However, despite taking them regularly his condition did not improve. The patient is reluctant to start clozapine. Which of the following drugs should be tried instead?

    A   Aripiprazole
    B   Chlorpromazine
    C   Flupenthixol decanoate injection
    D   Olanzapine
    E   Pipotiazine depot injection

33. What is the clinical effect of the occlusion of the stem of the posterior cerebral artery?

    A   Alexia in the visible field
    B   Contralateral ballism

      C   Cortical blindness +/– amnesia
      D   Homonymous hemianopia
      E   Ipsilateral third nerve palsy + contralateral hemiplegia

34. Which of the following is a key component of psychodynamic interpersonal therapy?

      A   Developing personal understanding
      B   Focus on change
      C   Focus on past and present
      D   Free floating
      E   Gaining better understanding of one's feelings

35. Which of the following antipsychotics has the least effect on serum prolactin levels?

      A   Amisulpride
      B   Chlorpromazine
      C   Haloperidol
      D   Olanzapine
      E   Risperidone

36. Which of the following activities is employed in psychodynamic psychotherapy?

      A   Activity scheduling and safe experiments
      B   Diaries and recoding of thoughts, feelings and behaviours
      C   Discussion about childhood experiences with a therapist, with exploration of 'slips of the tongue'
      D   Gradual exposure to anxiety-provoking situations with relaxation in a hierarchal fashion
      E   Rapid eye movements following an object while experiencing distressing thoughts

37. Which of the following information about chromosomal trisomy is correct?

      A   Abnormal chromosomal rearrangements
      B   Abnormal chromosomal deletions
      C   Abnormal chromosomal translocations
      D   Abnormal number of autosomes
      E   Abnormal number of sex chromosomes

38. A 44-year-old man with a family history of suicide presented with motor restlessness, slow saccadic eye movements, writhing movements of the protruded tongue and mild dysdiadochokinesia. What is the most likely diagnosis?

      A   Early onset Alzheimer's disease
      B   Huntington's disease
      C   Parkinson's disease
      D   Variant Creutzfeldt–Jakob disease
      E   Wilson's disease

39. Which of the following disorders is most closely associated with the defence mechanisms of isolation and undoing?

      A   Agoraphobia
      B   Anankastic-personality disorder
      C   Obsessive-compulsive disorder
      D   Panic disorder
      E   Social phobia

40. Which therapy involves circular questioning?

      A   Cognitive–analytical therapy

B   Family therapy
C   Interpersonal therapy
D   Multisystem therapy
E   Psychodynamic therapy

41. Which of the following statements about central nervous system axons is correct?

A   They are myelinated by Schwan cells
B   They contain axonal initial segment stems from the neuronal soma, which is devoid of Nissl's granules
C   They conduct towards the perikaryon
D   They contain Golgi complexes
E   They do not contain neurofilaments and microtubules

42. Which of the following antidepressants is available as an intravenous injection as well as an oral preparation in the UK?

A   Citalopram
B   Fluvoxamine
C   Fluoxetine
D   Paroxetine
E   Sertraline

43. Which of the following therapies is employed in the management of alcohol abuse, when the patient is presented with a small yet unpleasant electric shock immediately after consuming alcohol?

A   Assertiveness training
B   Aversion therapy
C   Flooding
D   Participant modelling
E   Stimulus control

44. Which of the following is a characteristic feature of axon myelination?

A   Complete before birth
B   No saltatory conduction
C   Performed by satellite cells in the peripheral nervous system
D   Precedes neuronal growth
E   Support regeneration of damaged peripheral nerves

45. A 27-year-old man's self-harm behaviour and substance misuse increased outside his therapy sessions when particularly difficult emotions were being addressed. Which term best describes this behaviour?

A   Acting out
B   Containment
C   Countertransference holding
D   Projection
E   Transference

46. Susceptibility alleles at a few genetic loci cause an increased risk of a disorder in an individual, although on their own they do not cause the disorder. What is this phenomenon called?

A   Genomic imprinting
B   Mitochondrial inheritance
C   Oligogenic inheritance
D   Polygenic inheritance
E   Quantitative trait locus inheritance

47. What part of the brain, when damaged, can cause homonymous hemianopia?

   A   Complete optic nerve
   B   Meyer's loop
   C   Optic chiasma
   D   Partial optic nerve
   E   Visual cortex

48. A 23-year-old woman had short stature, webbed neck, low hairline and a broad chest. Which of the following is the most likely diagnosis?

   A   Down's syndrome
   B   Edwards' syndrome
   C   Meta-female
   D   Patau's syndrome
   E   Turner's syndrome

49. The risk of certain mental illnesses is increased in first-degree relatives of patients with schizophrenia. However, you can reassure a relative of a patient with one of the conditions described below by stating that there is no increased risk with the following disorder. What is this disorder called?

   A   Bipolar affective disorder
   B   Paranoid personality disorder
   C   Persistent delusional disorder
   D   Schizoaffective disorder
   E   Schizotypal personality disorder

50. 'If I don't succeed, I must be a complete failure.' Of what thinking error, as described by Beck in his cognitive model, is this an example?

   A   All-or-nothing thinking
   B   Arbitrary inference
   C   Labelling
   D   Overgeneralisation
   E   Selective attention

51. Which of the following describes a fatal toxicity index?

   A   Number of cases in which toxic symptoms manifest per million prescriptions issued
   B   Number of cases of fetal or neonatal toxicity due to medication prescribed per million prescriptions issued
   C   Number of overdose deaths per million prescriptions issued
   D   Number of overdose deaths per 10,000 prescriptions issued
   E   Number of overdose deaths per 1000 prescriptions issued

52. Which of the following statements about gene characteristics is correct?

   A   A dominant allele, recessive allele, or both can manifest their effects in heterozygotes.
   B   Autosomal dominant disorders do not skip generations
   C   Autosomal recessive disorders do not remain hidden for several generations
   D   Disease genes are described as non-dominant or non-recessive
   E   In X-linked disorders, father-to-son transmission can take place

53. Which of the following is a characteristic feature of Williams' (Williams–Beuren) syndrome?

   A   Excessively hostile to strangers
   B   Learning disability is usually severe

C   Mild learning disability occurs in 75% of the patients
D   There are no cardiovascular anomalies
E   Williams' syndrome is caused by a chromosomal deletion at 7p11.23

54. Which nucleus of the thalamus is considered to be a part of the limbic system?

A   Anterior nucleus
B   Lateral nucleus
C   Medial nucleus
D   Posterior nucleus
E   Ventral nucleus

55. One of your patients was taking an antidepressant medication on her own. She informed you that she purchased this off the market. After some years, she had visual disturbance and was reported to have macular degeneration. Which of the following antidepressants is most likely to cause this?

A   Amitriptyline
B   Fluoxetine
C   Mirtazapine
D   Sertraline
E   St John's wort

56. Which of the following is the efferent from the cerebellar cortex?

A   Basket cells
B   Climbing fibre
C   Mossy fibre
D   Purkinje cells
E   Stellate cells

57. Which of the following are the largest cells of all neurons in the human brain?

A   Basket cells
B   Betz cells
C   Granule cells
D   Purkinje cells
E   Renshaw cells

58. What is the mechanism of caffeine's neuropsychiatric effects?

A   Adenosine receptor antagonism
B γ-Aminobutyric acid antagonism
C   Nicotinic acetylcholine receptor antagonism
D N-Methyl-D-aspartate antagonism
E   Opioid antagonism

59. How much of lithium is present in a 400-mg tablet of lithium carbonate?

A   0.5 mmol
B   5.4 mmol
C   6.8 mmol
D   10.8 mmol
E   12.2 mmol

60. What is the name of the fraction of individuals with a genotype in whom a disease could manifest?

A   Dominance
B   Expression

C   Manifestation
D   Penetrance
E   Visibility

61. Which of the following is 5-HT$_{2C}$-receptor antagonist?

A   Agomelatine
B   Mianserin
C   Quetiapine
D   Risperidone
E   Trazodone

62. Which of the following statements about epigenesis is correct?

A   Epigenesis is not an important consideration when behavioural phenotype is considered
B   Epigenesis refers to processes by which genes are affected by the phenotype
C   Epigenesis refers to the underlying processes by which the genotype gives rise to a phenotype
D   Failure of DNA oxidation in fragile X syndrome is an example of a deficit in epigenesis
E   Genetic imprinting is epinucleic

63. For what is sertindole licensed?

A   Anxiety
B   Depression
C   Mania
D   Schizophrenia
E   Tics

64. Which immune changes are seen in patients with depression?

A   Increased response of lymphocytes to mitogens
B   Lower natural killer cell activity
C   Lower acute phase reactants
D   Lower cytokine level
E   Lower expression of tryptophan oxygenase

65. Which of the following is the correct order in which the genes are expressed to form proteins?

A   Modifications of mRNA, transcription, translation and finally post-translational modifications of protein into its mature form
B   Transcription, modifications of mRNA, translation and finally post-translational modifications of protein into its mature form
C   Transcription, translation, modifications of mRNA and finally post-translational modifications of protein into its mature form
D   Translation, modifications of mRNA, transcription and finally transformation of protein into its mature form
E   Translation, post-translational modifications, transcription and transformation

66. Which of the following statements about fetal alcohol syndrome is correct?

A   Drinking 5 units/week is assumed to be safe in the mid to last trimester of pregnancy
B   Adaptive behaviour is usually well maintained in twins
C   Concordance rate for monozygotic and dizygotic twins is the same
D   Prevalence is 5.2:10,000 live births
E   There is only prenatal growth retardation

67. Which of the following is useful in the treatment of narcolepsy?

    A   Monoamine oxidase inhibitors
    B   Mirtazapine
    C   Selective serotonin reuptake inhibitors
    D   Tricyclic antidepressants
    E   Venlafaxine

68. Which of the following neurotransmitters does not activate c-*fos*?

    A   Acetylcholine
    B   Dopamine
    C γ-Aminobutyric acid
    D   Noradrenaline
    E   Serotonin

69. What is the close pairing of homologous chromosomes during the prophase stage of meiotic division called?

    A   Assembly
    B   Combination
    C   Linkage
    D   Recombination
    E   Synapsis

70. Which of the following conditions is caused by a trinucleotide (CAG) repeat?

    A   Fragile X syndrome
    B   Friedreich's ataxia
    C   Huntington's disease
    D   Myoclonic dystrophy
    E   Myoclonus epilepsy

71. Which of the following antidepressants is safe in patients with ventricular arrhythmias?

    A   Amitriptyline
    B   Clomipramine
    C   Desipramine
    D   Imipramine
    E   Lofepramine

72. Which of the following is the consequence of vitamin B_{12} deficiency?

    A   Megaloblastic anaemia
    B   Pellagra
    C   Peripheral and cranial nerve problems
    D   Subacute combined degeneration of the spinal cord
    E   Wernicke's encephalopathy

73. Which of the following conditions characterised by severe learning disability, microcephaly and cleft lip is caused by chromosome 13 trisomy?

    A   Down's syndrome
    B   Edwards' syndrome
    C   Patau's syndrome
    D   Meta-female
    E   Turner's syndrome

74. Which of the lysosomal disorders is correctly matched with its corresponding enzyme deficiency?

    A   Gaucher's disease: galactocerebroside β-galactosidase
    B   Hurler's syndrome: hexosaminidase
    C   Metachromatic leukodystrophy: arylsulphatase A deficiency
    D   Niemann–Pick disease: α_1-iduronidase
    E   Tay–Sachs disease: sphingomyelinase

75. In relation to schizophrenia, the model of multifocal inheritance assumes that two or more genes at different loci act together, resulting in a clinical phenotype. What is this concept called?

    A   Co-factor
    B   Dominant
    C   Epigenetics
    D   Epistasis
    E   Epithetic

76. Which of the following is a long QTc syndrome?

    A   Brugada's syndrome
    B   DiGeorge's syndrome
    C   Dressler's syndrome
    D   Romano–Ward syndrome
    E   Wolf–Parkinson–White syndrome

77. In which of the following phases of cell cycle does cell division take place?

    A   G0 phase
    B   G1 phase
    C   G2 phase
    D   M Phase
    E   S phase

78. Which of the following statements about the Prader–Willi syndrome is correct?

    A   Compulsive eating is limited to specific foods/eatables/drinks
    B   Compulsive eating is the most disabling behaviour
    C   Hypogonadism is least useful for diagnosis during and after adolescence
    D   It occurs as a result of paternal deletion of 15q11-q21 or maternal uniparental disomy of chromosome 15 or an imprinting centre mutation
    E   Self-cutting is the most common form of self-injury found in around 20%

79. With regards to learning disabilities (LDs), which of the following statements is correct?

    A   Abnormalities of the autosomal chromosomes usually cause no anatomical deformities
    B   Abnormalities of the autosomal chromosomes usually cause mild LDs
    C   Abnormalities of the autosomal chromosomes usually cause severe LDs with widespread anatomical deformities
    D   Abnormalities of the autosomal chromosomes usually cause severe LDs with no anatomical deformities
    E   Sex chromosome abnormalities are always associated with LDs

80. Which of the following is responsible for formation of the hippocampus?

    A   Amygdaloid nucleus
    B   Corpus striatum
    C   Cingulate gyrus
    D   Dentate gyrus
    E   Visual association cortex

81. A 30-year-old man presented with learning disability, Lisch nodules in the eyes and intracranial tumours. What is the most likely diagnosis?

    A   Ataxia telangiectasia
    B   Tuberous sclerosis
    C   Sturge–Weber syndrome
    D   Von Hippel–Lindau disease
    E   Von Recklinghausen's neurofibromatosis

82. Which of the following describes the differences between variant Creutzfeldt–Jakob disease (vCJD) and sporadic Creutzfeldt–Jakob disease (sCJD)?

    A   Electroencephalography (EEG) and cerebrospinal fluid examination are more useful in vCJD in sCJD
    B   Tonsillar biopsy is negative in vCJD
    C   Typical EEG changes are seen in vCJD
    D   Variant CJD has an earlier onset of illness than sCJD
    E   Variant CJD is more common than sCJD

83. Which of the following cranial nerves supplies the intrinsic muscles of the tongue?

    A   Accessory nerve
    B   Glossopharyngeal nerve
    C   Hypoglossal nerve
    D   Vagus nerve
    E   Vestibulocochlear nerve

84. Which of the following genetic defects is seen in Down's syndrome?

    A   Chimera
    B   Duplication
    C   Meiotic arrest
    D   Robertsonian translocation
    E   Translocation

85. Which of the following statements about Turner's syndrome is correct?

    A   Imprinted genes affect the brain's structure and function
    B   It is commonly associated with intellectual disability
    C   It is associated with one Barr body
    D   The 'X' chromosome in 'XO' is derived from the mother
    E   The 'X' chromosome in 'XO' is derived from the father

86. Which of the following is the third messenger?

    A   Calcium
    B   Cyclic AMP
    C   c-*fos*
    D   CREB (cAMP response element-binding protein)
    E   Serotonin

87. Which of the following cerebral tumours derive from blood vessels?

    A   Gliomas
    B   Haemangioblastomas
    C   Pituitary adenomas
    D   Medulloblastomas
    E   Meningeal tumours

88. Which of the following structures is part of the occipital lobe?

    A   Amygdaloid nucleus
    B   Corpus striatum
    C   Cingulate gyrus
    D   Dentate gyrus
    E   Visual association cortex

89. Which of the following is commonly seen in patients with tardive dyskinesia?

    A   Increased levels of homovanillic acid
    B   Increased levels of homovanillic acid in plasma
    C   Increased prolactin levels
    D   Increased urinary homovanillic acid levels
    E   Presence of lipid peroxidation byproduct in blood

90. Which of the following structures contains anterior cingulate cortex?

    A   Dorsolateral prefrontal cortex
    B   Frontal operculum
    C   Inferior mesial region
    D   Superior mesial region
    E   Superior temporal gyrus

91. Which of the following features is found in post-stroke patients?

    A   Evocation of thoughts
    B   Forced thinking
    C   Panoramic memory
    D   Pathological crying
    E   Uncinate crisis

92. Which of these is a method employed to distinguish genetic influence from common environmental effects that contribute to aggregation of disease in families?

    A   Association studies
    B   Allele-sharing methods
    C   Linkage disequilibrium in analysis
    D   Path analysis
    E   Twin studies

93. Which of the following tests is used to detect, localise brain lesions and determine their effects?

    A   Bender's visual motor gestalt test
    B   Halstead–Reitan battery
    C   Luria–Nebraska neuropsychological battery
    D   Cambridge neuropsychological test automated battery
    E   Wechsler's adult intelligence scale

94. In which phase of meiosis does recombination take place?

    A   Metaphase I
    B   Metaphase II
    C   Prophase I
    D   Prophase II
    E   Interphase

95. Which of the following is consistent with human DNA characteristics?

    A   It is less than 2 metres long
    B   It contains approximately 3.9×10^9 base-pairs
    C   Total DNA complement in a cell is called a gene
    D   97% of a genome consists of the coding sequence
    E   2–3% of a genome has no apparent function

96. In mammalian chromosome replication, approximately what numbers of nucleotides are added per minute?

    A   30
    B   300
    C   3000
    D   30,000
    E   300,000

97. Which of the following statements about Lesch–Nyhan disease is correct?

    A   Ambivalent statements and coprolalia are characteristic features
    B   It is an autosomal recessive disease
    C   It is an acquired error of purine nucleotide metabolism
    D   Its occurrence in males and females is usually the same
    E   The patients usually have severe intellectual disability

98. Which of the following is related to narcolepsy?

    A   Cholecystokinin
    B   Neurotensin
    C   Opioid neuropeptide
    D   Orexin
    E   Substance P

99. Which of the following structures contains a supplementary motor area?

    A   Dorsolateral prefrontal cortex
    B   Frontal operculum
    C   Inferior mesial region
    D   Superior mesial region
    E   Superior temporal gyrus

100. In which of the following is an increased level of homovanillic acid found?

    A   Adrenal medullary tumour
    B   Bulimia nervosa
    C   Parkinson's disease
    D   Schizophrenia
    E   Severe depression

101. Which of the following pairs about dementia and EEG changes is correctly matched?

    A   Alzheimer's dementia: diffuse slowing of α rhythm
    B   Frontotemporal dementia: focal slow activity in temporal region
    C   Lewy body dementia: increased fast activity wave rhythm
    D   Peudodementia: periodic sharp waves
    E   Vascular dementi: initial loss of α waves

102. Although nuclear DNA is most important, another cell organelle containing DNA mainly inherited through the female lineage is vital. Which of the following is this cell organelle?

   A   Endoplasmic reticulum
   B   Golgi apparatus
   C   Mitochondria
   D   Plasma membrane
   E   Ribosomes

103. To what does a group of conditions that are necessary to provide adequate evidence of a causal relationship between an incidence and a consequence refer?

   A   Attributable risk
   B   Bradford Hill criteria
   C   Counter factual consideration
   D   Persistence
   E   Population-attributable risk

104. The association between Alzheimer's disease and Down's syndrome assisted the detection of linkage of familial Alzheimer's disease on chromosome 21. What does this describe?

   A   Candidate gene approach
   B   Hybridisation
   C   Positional cloning
   D   Position effect
   E   Translocation

105. At what level is gene expression primarily controlled at?

   A   DNA methylation
   B   Genetic linkage
   C   Post-translational processing
   D   Transcription
   E   Translation

106. Which of the following statements about Down's syndrome is correct?

   A   Congenital heart malformations are present in 50% of patients with Down's syndrome
   B   Early deaths are associated with associated congenital anomalies, especially hypothyroidism
   C   In 1960, Down gave the first description of the syndrome now known as Down's syndrome
   D   It was the first syndrome in which a sex-chromosomal anomaly was demonstrated as the basis of characteristic physical features
   E   The underlying genetic abnormality (trisomy 21) was identified in 1980

107. What is the mutation of a single gene resulting in a disease with a wide range of symptoms called?

   A   Isotropic
   B   Monogenic
   C   Pleiotropism
   D   Polygenic
   E   Polytrophic

108. Which of the following statements about dementia in Down's syndrome is correct?

   A   The ε2 allele is associated with an increased risk of dementia
   B   Evidence of dementia is found in 100% of patients after 50 years of age
   C   Frontotemporal dementia is the most common dementia in Down's syndrome

D A high risk for dementia in adults with Down's syndrome has been linked to triplication and overexpression of the gene for amyloid precursor protein

E There is delayed onset of menopause and dementia in women

109. At which stage of cell division does recombination (also known as crossover) of genetic material occur?

A Anaphase stage of mitotic division

B Anaphase stage of meiotic division

C Metaphase stage of meiotic division

D Prophase of mitotic division

E Prophase stage of meiosis division

110. Velocardiofacial syndrome (VCSF) or Shprintzen's syndrome has an estimated prevalence of 1:3000, i.e. second most common genetic syndrome after Down's syndrome. Which of the following statements about VCSF is correct?

A The 22q11.4 syndrome includes VCSF and DiGeorge's syndrome

B It is inherited as an autosomal recessive condition

C It is denoted as a 22q11.4 deletion syndrome

D Offspring of an individual with deletion of 22q11.2 syndrome have a 50% chance of inheriting the 22q11.2 deletion

E The psychotic and affective symptoms emerge only in adulthood

111. Which of the following is an example of chromosomal monosomy?

A 45,X

B 46,XX

C 47,XY + 21

D 69,XXY

E 92,XXYY

112. The 5 mL dose of 509 mg/5 mL oral solution of lithium citrate is equivalent to how many milligrams of lithium carbonate?

A 100

B 200

C 300

D 400

E 500

113. What is the number of new cases of a disease occurring per year called?

A Additional rate

B Attritional rate

C Incidence

D Insolence

E Prevalence

114. Which of the following is correct with regard to catecholamine-O-methyl transferase?

A Affecting the N-methyl-D-aspartate receptor modulator D-serine

B Glutamate release

C Multiple roles in glutamate signalling

D Regulating function of dopamine in the frontal cortex

E Synaptic signalling

115. In which of the following conditions are senile plaques seen?

    A   Down's syndrome
    B   Dementia pugilistica
    C   Lytico–Bodig disease
    D   Postencephalitic Parkinson's disease
    E   Progressive supranuclear palsy

116. From where does an anterior thalamic nucleus receive its efferents?

    A   Cingulate gyrus
    B   Prefrontal cortex
    C   Motor cortex
    D   Primary auditory cortex
    E   Supplementary motor area

Answers: MCQs

1. A Down's syndrome

Most cases of Down's syndrome are caused by trisomy of chromosome 21. This results from non-disjunction during meiosis and accounts for about 95% cases of Down's syndrome. Edwards' syndrome is due to trisomy of chromosome 18, Patau's syndrome is caused by trisomy of chromosome 13, Turner's syndrome is due to a single X chromosome and meta-female is trisomy of the X chromosome.

2. B Death of a loved one

Interpersonal therapy developed by Klerman and Weissman addresses four interpersonal problem areas such as:

1. Grief
2. Interpersonal role disputes
3. Role transitions
4. Interpersonal deficits.

It deals with problems in the present context and lasts for 12–16 weeks.

3. B Penicillamine

This young man most probably has Wilson's disease. Progressive hepatolenticular degeneration, or Wilson's disease, is a genetic disorder of copper metabolism. It is characterised by psychiatric (e.g. depression, anxiety and psychosis) and neurological symptoms (e.g. parkinsonism, ataxia and choreoathetoid movements) at a young age. Decreased serum ceruloplasmin and increased urinary copper usually confirm the diagnosis; however, liver biopsy is the most definitive investigation. Penicillamine, a chelating agent, is the drug of choice. Tetrabenazine is indicated for Huntington's disease and tardive dyskinesia. Benztropine is an anticholinergic used to manage antipsychotic medication side effects.

4. D Tetrabenazine

This is licensed in the UK for treatment of tardive dyskinesia. Several other agents have been tried with mixed success, supported by clinical experience, small studies, case reports, etc. These include benzodiazepines, vitamin E, amino acids, botulinum toxin, calcium antagonists, pyridoxine, naltrexone, and many others. Besides tetrabenazine, benzodiazepines and vitamin E have the most literature but evidence is far from conclusive. Tetrabenazine is used at a dose of 25–200 mg/day.

5. E Posteroinferior cerebellar artery

The lateral medullary syndrome is caused by thrombosis of the vertebral artery and posteroinferior cerebellar artery in the lateral part of the medulla. The clinical picture depends on the extent to which the related nuclei and pathways are damaged. The symptoms may be vertigo, vomiting, dysphagia, nystagmus, cerebellar ataxia and hoarseness, Horner's syndrome (ptosis, anhidrosis, and miosis) and cross-pattern sensory loss.

6. D There is deletion of chromosome 11, and it presents with aniridia, reduced IQ and ambiguous genitalia

WAGR stands for Wilms' tumour, aniridia, genitourinary anomalies and learning disability (mental retardation).

Deletion on the short arm of chromosome 5 is called cri-du-chat syndrome when the child presents with craniofacial abnormalities, microcephaly, learning disability and abnormal cry. Deletion on the long arm of paternal chromosome 15 is called Prader–Willi syndrome and presents with reduced height, smaller hands, feet and testicles, infantile hypotonia and angry outbursts. There is a deletion on chromosome 13 which can lead to bilateral retinoblastoma with reduced IQ.

Jacobsen's syndrome is due to loss of genetic material on the long (q) arm of chromosome 11. It is also called 11q terminal deletion disorder. The patient would have delayed developmental milestones such as sitting, standing, walking. Speech is also delayed with cognitive impairment and learning difficulties. Due to their behavioural problems, many people with Jacobsen's syndrome are usually diagnosed with attention deficit hyperactivity disorder. It manifests with typical facial features, which are a broad nasal bridge, small low-set ears, widely set eyes, drooping eyelids, epicanthal folds and a small lower jaw. Affected individuals often have a large head, which gives the forehead a pointed appearance of the forehead, called trigonocephaly.

7. D Psychodrama

This was developed by Moreno and involves group therapy and use of special dramatic methods. The following are explored by psychodrama:

- Personality constitution
- Interpersonal relationships
- Conflicts
- Emotional problems.

The following roles are employed by psychodrama: director, protagonist, auxiliary ego and group.

8. E Tonsillar biopsy

It is the most sensitive and specific diagnostic procedure for variant Creutzfeldt–Jakob disease (CJD). Human PrP gene (PRNP) is analysed in the inherited CJD. MRI especially fluid-attenuated inversion recovery (FLAIR) sequence is the most useful non-invasive neuroimaging technique in the advanced stage of variant CJD. There is a bilateral increased signal in the posterior thalamus, known as the pulvinar sign. The electroencephalography in variant CJD shows generalised slowing with no pseudoperiodic pattern, which is found in sporadic CJD. The PrPSc type is detected on western blot in variant CJD.

9. D Frataxin

Trinucleotide repeats occur in many disorders that have a mental health phenotype. The repetitions can be different such as (CGC) >200 for fragile X syndrome and (GAA) 7–200 in Friedreich's ataxia. The repetitions change the protein code and the cells have a loss of function.

10. B Emergence of latent meanings

The modern view of transference is the emergency of latent meaning that is brought on by the intensity of the relationship between patient and analyst.

The classic view of transference is that the patient transfers onto the analyst strong feelings from past experiences that were previously experienced as a child.

Other options are definitions of countertransference:

- Affective resonance and empathy: Stern, Winnicott
- The results of projective identification: Klein, Bion, Steiner
- Part of the bipersonal or intersubjective field: Sullivan, Langs
- The analyst's blind spot or resistance: Freud, Sandler.

11. B Haloperidol

This belongs to the class of butyrophenones. In 1958, when Janssen laboratories were trying to create a stronger analgesic, haloperidol was created as a byproduct of pethidine. Chlorpromazine is a chlorinated derivative of promazine. Trifluoperazine is synthesised by alkylation of 2-trifluoromethyl-phenothiazine-4-methyl-1-piperazinyl propyl chloride. Thioridazine is synthesised by alkylating 2-methylthiophenothiazine with 2-(2-chloroethyl)-1-methylpiperidine. Risperidone is a benzoxazole derivative.

12. E Thalamus

This is the largest nuclear mass in the entire nervous system. All the thalamic nuclei except the reticular nucleus have reciprocal excitatory connection with the cerebral cortex. They are categorised into three functional groups, i.e. specific nuclei, association nuclei and non-specific nuclei. The specific nuclei are related to specific motor or sensory area of the cerebral cortex. The association nuclei are reciprocally connected to the associations of the cerebral cortex. The non-specific nuclei are not specific to any one sensory modality.

13. A Brewin

He proposed that two main memory systems are essential for our understanding of post-traumatic stress disorder. These include: verbally accessible, declarative memory and situationally accessible non-declarative memory.

14. C Left hippocampal density

In chronically depressed patients, it has been shown that there was temporal enlargement and left hippocampal density was associated with delayed verbal recognition.

15. A Displacement

According to Vaillant, defence mechanisms can be classed in hierarchy. A person's defences may shift depending on life stressors.

Table 5.1 Classification of ego defence mechanisms	
Hierarchy	Types
Mature	Anticipation and objectivity, suppression, altruism, sublimation, humour
Intermediate	Repression, reaction formation, displacement
Immature	Passive aggression, hypochondriasis, 'acting out', dissociation, projection, schizoid fantasy
Primitive	Splitting, delusional projection, denial

16. A Gaze aversion is a very noticeable feature of fragile X syndrome

There are certain characteristic behavioural phenotypes that, when present in individuals with known chromosomal, genetic or neurodevelopmental disorders, will suggest the presence of the syndrome: hyperphagia and compulsive behaviour in Prader–Willi syndrome; self-mutilation of fingers and lips in Lesch–Nyhan syndrome; hand and hand to mouth stereotypies in Rett's syndrome. Behavioural phenotypes are stereotypical patterns of behaviour that are reliably identified in groups of individuals with known neurodevelopmental disorders and are 'not learned'. As Nyhan suggested, these are 'syndromes of behaviour' after he observed self-injurious behaviour to be so common in Lesch–Nyhan syndrome when he introduced the term 'behavioural phenotype'. Superficial sociability, hyperlalia and language disorder are present in Williams' syndrome.

17. A Countertransference

During psychoanalysis, there are times when the patient evokes certain emotions in the therapist. Originally Freud considered this to be an obstacle. However, more recently, this process in which an analyst experiences emotions that are projected onto them by the patient is considered to be a therapeutic tool, termed 'countertransference'; it reveals information about the patient's internal object world.

18. A Catecholamine hydroxylase gene

Neuregulin, dysbindin and disrupted-in-schizophrenia 1 (DISC1) are the commonest genes isolated in relation to schizophrenia. Catecholamine-O-methyl transferase has been found in association studies and G72 (D-amino acid oxidase activator [DAOA]) in linkage studies have been associated with schizophrenia G72 (DAOA).

19. B Haloperidol

Haloperidol and trifluoperazine are licensed for use in children. However, they have a lot of extrapyramidal side effects. Most of the newer antipsychotics are not licensed for use in children. Aripiprazole is not licensed for use in children <15 years of age, and also not licensed for treating mania in children. Risperidone is not licensed for use in children <15 years of age for psychoses and also not licensed for treating autism in children. Quetiapine and olanzapine are not licensed for treating psychoses in children.

20. E Poor frustration tolerance

The primary aim of supportive psychotherapy is to support reality testing, provide ego support and attempt to re-establish the level of functioning. It is employed in otherwise healthy individuals with on-going crises. It is useful in those who are not psychologically motivated to 'explore' themselves. The therapy is not time limited and the therapist must be predictable and available in times of need.

21. A Conduction dysphasis

This occurs due to damage to the arcuate fasciculus which connects Wernicke's area to premotor and motor areas. Previously it was believed that it connected Broca's area anteriorly to Wernicke's area posteriorly, but research has shown otherwise. If the arcuate fasciculus is damaged, patients struggle with heard speech; however, they are able to comprehend speech.

22. B Cannabis

Symptoms of cannabis (cannabis flashbacks) use may also occur days or weeks after high-dose consumption of cannabis. It is rare and requires a personal vulnerability or may be because of interaction of cannabis with other drugs.

23. D Phase 4 clinical trials

The cost utility of the latest antipsychotic drugs in schizophrenia study (CUtLASS) and the clinical antipsychotic trials of intervention effectiveness (CATIE) were comparative studies of different antipsychotics from the first and second generation. They followed up these patients for a period of time to assess cost utility and effectiveness. These studies found few differences in effectiveness between first-generation antipsychotics (FGAs) and second-generation antipsychotics (SGAs) in non-refractory patients. They are examples of phase 4 clinical trials. Phase 1 trials are done in healthy volunteers to see the tolerability and side effects of the drug. Phase 2 studies help to determine the optimal dose range. Some phase 2 studies are efficacy studies. Phase 4 studies are post-marketing surveillance studies.

24. A Accept themselves and others for what they are

Maslow believed that certain behaviours could lead one to become self-actualising. He advocated experiencing life as a child does and to listen to your own feelings in evaluating experiences: be honest, assume responsibility and be prepared to be unpopular. Work hard at whatever you do and try to identify your own defences and have the courage to give them up. Self-actualisers have deep appreciation of basic experiences in life.

Some of the characteristics of self-actualisers are:

- Acceptance and realism: realistic perceptions of themselves, others and the world around them
- Problem centring: concerned with problem solving outside themselves, motivated by a sense of personal responsibility and ethics
- Spontaneity: spontaneous in thoughts and behaviour
- Autonomy and solitude: enjoy company of others but also need time to focus on self-development
- Continued appreciation
- Peak experience: often have experiences of intense joy, wonder and awe.

25. B Bion

Winifred Bion developed the idea of containment, suggesting that, for individuals to develop coherent ways of representing relationships between self and other, and for thinking about the content of their own mind, they need to develop within a particular interpersonal setting.

26. D Ophidiophobia

Arachnophobia is a phobia of spiders.

Table 5.2 Classification of phobias	
Phobias	**Specific phobias**
Arachnophobia	Spiders
Cyanophobia	Blue colour
Cynophobia	Dogs
Herpetophobia	Reptiles
Ophidiophobia	Snakes
Zemmiphobia	Rats

27. B Emotional circuit

Basal ganglia involve the striatum, pallidum, subthalamic nucleus and compact part of substantia nigra. There are at least four circuits that start in the cerebral cortex, traverse the basal ganglion and return to the cortex. They are the motor loop, cognitive loop, limbic loop and oculomotor loop. The amygdala is primarily associated with the emotion of fear.

28. D They have DNA segments that does not code for amino acids called exons

There are around 100,000 human genes in the human genome. A gene is a segment of DNA encoding for a single/limited set of proteins. The alternative forms of the same gene are called alleles. Each gene has two alleles; a person is said to homozygous in respect of that gene if the two alleles are same, and if they differ the individual is said to be heterozygous. Genes make up only for 1% of the total human DNA. The remainder is for regulatory and supportive purpose. Within genes there are segments of DNA that do not code for amino acids. These are called introns (they remain inside the nucleus) whereas exons are DNA segments that are transported into the cytoplasm and they code for amino acids.

29. D Reformulation, revision and recognition

During cognitive–analytical therapy, reformulation is the first step of the above three. This step happens around the fourth to fifth session. The objective of reformulation is to understand association between past experiences and presenting problems. Recognition is the next step in the process in which unhelpful procedures are identified. It is crucial that these unhelpful methods be identified before new methods can be devised. This is known as revision and is the final phase of the three mentioned in the question.

30. E Sensation

The gestalt awareness cycle includes the following stages: contract, satisfaction, withdrawal, sensation, awareness, mobilisation and action.

31. B Clonus

Sudden interruption of the corticospinal tract is characterised by the following features:

- Initial flaccid paralysis with loss of tendon reflexes
- Spasticity with abnormally brisk reflexes.

Clonus can often be elicited. Babinski's sign is positive and abdominal reflexes are absent on the affected side.

32. D Olanzapine

It is sensible to think about using a depot antipsychotic in a patient in whom compliance is an issue. Clinical antipsychotic trials of intervention effectiveness study showed that, in patients who tried and failed on the first atypical antipsychotic, switching to olanzapine or risperidone was associated with better outcome than switching to quetiapine or ziprasidone. The Maudsley guidance suggests that, if a patient has not tried on olanzapine or risperidone yet, it would be a reasonable decision to switch to these drugs provided that the side-effect balance is favourable.

33. D Homonymous hemianopia

This is caused by occlusion of either stem. Alexia in the visible field is caused by left stem occlusion. Cortical blindness with or without amnesia is caused by occlusion of both stems. Contralateral ballism is caused by occlusion in the subthalamic nucleus branch of the posterior cerebral artery.

34. B Focus on change

Hobson developed psychodynamic interpersonal therapy and gave the key components as:

- Rationale for exploratory therapy
- Developing a shared understanding
- Focus on the here and now
- Gaining better understanding of interpersonal problems
- Structure
- Focus on change.

35. D Olanzapine

Many antipsychotics can cause an increase in the serum prolactin levels. Exceptions include aripiprazole, clozapine, olanzapine, quetiapine and ziprasidone.

36. C Discussion about childhood experiences with a therapist, with exploration of 'slips of the tongue'

Psychodynamic work employs dream work and exploring parapraxis (slip of the tongue). The therapy explores the unconscious mind and helps to address difficulties experienced in early childhood.

37. D Abnormal number of autosomes

Trisomy is an abnormal number of autosomes. The commonest trisomy is Down's syndrome (trisomy 21), Edwards' syndrome (trisomy 18) and Patau's syndrome (trisomy 13).

38. B Huntington's disease

Patients with Huntington's disease (HD) attend a psychiatrist with initial complaints of depression, anxiety, irritability, psychosis, etc. These symptoms might be the only presentation for many years. The patient is at higher risk of suicide during this prodromal phase. Cognitive problems and irritability are usually out of proportion relative to other symptoms. Of the HD patients who present with schizophrenic symptoms, most are adolescents, and they may continue to present with psychosis and loss of cognitive efficiency for several years before presenting with motor symptoms. Children with HD often have grand mal seizures. A family history is usually positive and depression and suicide are commoner than in general population.

39. C Obsessive–compulsive disorder

Isolation, magical undoing and reaction formation are all associated with the psychodynamic understanding of obsessive–compulsive disorder. Magical thinking has at its core omnipotence of thought. The person believes that merely by thinking about an event in the external world he or she can cause the event to occur without intermediate physical actions. This feeling causes fear of aggressive thoughts.

40. B Family therapy

Circular and reflective questioning is employed in the Milan systemic family therapy. Here the various family members are questioned on their individual beliefs and perceptions about relationships. Asking each to comment and reflect on the answers given by the other family members creates feedback which allows for changes in the dynamics and interactions.

41. D Contain Golgi complexes

In the central nervous system, almost all the neurons are multipolar. Their cell bodies or soma has multiple poles with dendrites. The remaining part of the soma gives rise to axons. Most axons give off collateral branches. Most synaptic contacts are either axodendritic (excitatory) or axosomatic (inhibitory). All parts of the neuron are permeated by microtubules and neurofilaments. The soma contains the nucleus and perikaryon (cytoplasm). The perikaryon contains Golgi complexes and Nissl's bodies, which are clumps of granular endoplasmic reticulum.

42. A Citalopram

The only selective serotonin reuptake inhibitor available in intravenous and oral formulation is citalopram 40 mg/mL injection. Mirtazapine is also available as an intravenous preparation. Amitriptyline is available as an intramuscular and intravenous preparation. Clomipramine is available as an intravenous formulation.

Fluoxetine liquid has been tried as a sublingual formulation.

43. B Aversion therapy

This is commonly employed in the management of paraphilias and alcohol dependence. Here, after a specific behavioural response the individual is presented with an unpleasant noxious stimulus which acts as a punishment. This inhibits and is eventually extinguished. Examples of stimuli are electric shocks or corporal punishment. A series of sequences of the pairing of the unpleasant stimulus with the behaviour will result in the reduction and eventual abolishment of the unwanted behaviour.

44. E Support regeneration of damaged peripheral nerves

Myelination commences during the middle period of gestation and continues well into the second decade. In the central nervous system, myelination is carried out by oligodendrocytes and in the peripheral nervous system by Schwann cells. Myelination greatly increases the rate of impulse.

45. A Acting out

This is the way of expressing the unconscious fantasy impulsively through behaviour, and is the direct expression of an unconscious impulse. It is seen in patients with a personality disorder and examples include tantrums, self-harm behaviour and illicit substance misuse. This behaviour occurs outside the individual's reflective awareness and is considered by observers to be unaccompanied by guilt. It is important for clinicians to recognise and address.

46. C Oligogenic inheritance

This is an example of an e4 allele in apoE in Alzheimer's disease. Polygenic inheritance involves a combination of multiple additive genetic effects, and their interaction with environmental factors to cause complex disorders. Quantitative trait locus describes genes that basically contribute to continuously distributed traits. Genomic imprinting is the phenomenon whereby there is a difference of expression of genes, depending on whether the chromosomes are from the maternal or the paternal side. Mitochondria have mtDNA and mitochondrial inheritance follows a 'maternal inheritance pattern' because mitochondria are abundant in maternal eggs. Various disorders of muscle tissue and nervous tissue, mainly the optic nerve pathway such as in Leber's hereditary optic neuropathy, chronic progressive external ophthalmoplegia, are inherited via the mitochondrial genome.

47. E Visual cortex

A lesion in the partial optic nerve leads to ipsilateral scotoma.

A lesion in the complete optic nerve leads to blindness in that eye.

A lesion in the optic chiasma leads to bitemporal hemianopia.

A lesion in the optic tract leads to homonymous hemianopia.

A lesion in Meyer's loop leads to homonymous upper quadrantanopia.

Lesion in the optic radiation and visual cortex leads to homonymous hemianopia.

Lesion in the bilateral macular cortex leads to bilateral central scotomas.

48. E Turner's syndrome

This is caused by a sex chromosome abnormality. The phenotypic females have the genotype of 45X. The features of Turner's syndrome are low hairline, short stature, broad chest, webbed neck, and increased carrying angle, failure of breast development and lack of pubic hairs. The IQ level of these females is either comparable to the general population or lower by a mean of 10 points.

49. A Bipolar affective disorder

In a patient with schizophrenia, there is an increased risk of schizophrenia, schizoaffective disorder and schizotypal personality disorder in first-degree relatives. In patients with schizoaffective disorder, the risk of schizophrenia and a mood disorder is increased in first-degree relatives. The risk of bipolar affective disorder is not increased in first-degree relatives.

Stein G, Wilkinson G. Seminars in Adult Psychiatry, 2nd edn. London: Gaskell, 2007: 282.

50. A All-or-nothing thinking

The patient sees everything in black and white, missing all the shades of grey in between. In depression, this could lead to the above example.

The others include:

- Labelling is a global distortion and an overgeneralised negative view of the self. The patient labels him- or herself as hopeless, incompetent or a victim.
- Overgeneralisation is predicting a never-ending pattern of loss or defeat from a single event.
- Selective attention refers to remembering only the negative aspects and focusing selectively on them.
- Arbitrary inference is jumping to conclusions without looking at the evidence available.

51. C Number of overdose deaths per million prescriptions issued

Fatal toxicity index (FTI) is a measure of the number of overdose deaths per million prescriptions issued. FTI figures suggest high toxicity for tricyclic drugs (especially dosulepin but not lofepramine), medium toxicity for venlafaxine and moclobemide, and low toxicity for selective serotonin reuptake inhibitors, mirtazapine and reboxetine.

52. B Autosomal dominant disorders do not skip generations

Disease genes are described as dominant or recessive. A dominant allele will express itself in a heterozygous state but a recessive allele can express itself only in a homozygous state. In autosomal dominant (AD) disorders, unaffected: affected offspring ratio is 1:1. AD disorders do not skip generations. In autosomal recessive (AR) disorders, both parents are unaffected heterozygous carriers. Unaffected: affected offspring in AR is thus 3:1. Most X- linked disorders are recessive which is why the heterozygous females are unaffected. In X-linked recessive disorders, 50% of the sons are affected and 50% of the daughters are carriers. Father-to-son transmission does not take place in X-linked traits because the father passes only the Y chromosome to the son.

53. C Mild learning disability occurs in 75% of the patients

Williams' syndrome, which is caused by a chromosomal deletion at 7q11.23, presents with supravalvular aortic stenosis, pulmonary stenosis, mild intellectual disability in around 75% and unusual facial experience. A prenatal chorionic villous sampling at 10–12 weeks or amniocentesis at 16–18 weeks of gestation can help in detecting it prenatally. Excessive sociability and friendliness are present. Williams' syndrome is characterised by specific neuromorphological and neurophysiological findings on neuroimaging. MRI shows a proportional sparing of frontal, limbic and neocerebellar structures. *LIM-kinase1* and *STX1A* are the candidate genes for behavioural and cognitive function in this syndrome.

54. A Anterior nucleus is considered to be a part of the limbic system

55. E St John's wort

This contains a red pigment that can cause photosensitivity reactions. Hypericin may be phototoxic to the retina and can contribute to early development of macular degeneration. Fluoxetine, sertraline and mirtazapine are safe in this aspect. Amitriptyline can increase intraocular pressure and cause glaucoma. Hence careful monitoring is needed in susceptible patients.

56. D Purkinje cell

Purkinje cells are the only efferent (output) from the cerebellar cortex. Two kinds of fibres, climbing fibres from the inferior olivary nucleus and the mossy fibres from all other sources, are afferent (input) to the cerebellar cortex.

57. B Betz cells

They are the largest cells of all neurons in the human brain.

Purkinje cells are the largest of all cells in the cerebellum.

Golgi cells are the smallest of all cells in the cerebellum.

58. A Adenosine receptor antagonism

The main action of caffeine is antagonism of adenosine A_1- and A_2-receptors. Higher doses also block phosphodiesterase and γ-aminobutyric acid A.

Table 5.3 Mechanism of action of psychotropic drugs	
Receptor antagonism	Examples
N-Methyl-D-aspartate antagonism	Amantadine, ketamine, ethanol, riluzole
γ-Aminobutyric acid antagonism	Flumazenil
Nicotinic acetylcholinesterase antagonism	Nicotine
Opioid antagonism	Naloxone, naltrexone

59. D 10.8 mmol

Lithium carbonate 200 mg, 250 mg, 400 mg and 450 mg contains 5.4, 6.8, 10.8 and 12.2 mmol lithium respectively.

60. D Penetrance

The occurrence of clinical phenotype in a population carrying a genotype or defective gene is called penetrance. It is an all-or-none phenomenon. For example, Huntington's disease patients have high penetrance.

61. A Agomelatine

Other drugs that are 5-HT$_{2C}$-receptor antagonists:

Clozapine
Olanzapine
Mirtazapine
Doxepin

Other mentioned drugs: risperidone, quetiapine, trazodone and mianserin block 5-HT$_{2A}$-receptors.

62. C Epigenesis refers to the underlying processes by which the genotype gives rise to a phenotype

The term 'epigenetic' was introduced by Waddington in 1939 to describe the processes that constitute the pathways from genes to cognition and complex behaviour. This requires an understanding of the ways in which genes are controlled and direct the epigenetic programme. Epigenesis is a very important consideration when behavioural phenotype is considered.

Methylation is epinucleic and the failure of DNA methylation in fragile X syndrome is an example of a deficit in this type of epigenesis.

Any physical expression of a gene, i.e. the phenotype, is due to the DNA sequencing in the gene. Epigenesis is the study of the processes by which the change in heritable phenotype, i.e. changes in physical appearance, occur due to mechanisms other than the gene expression or changes in DNA sequence.

63. D Schizophrenia

Sertindole is licensed to be used in the treatment of schizophrenia. The initiation dose is 4 mg and the usual maintenance dose is 12–24 mg. The medication was limited and reintroduced in 2002 in Europe under strict monitoring. It was withdrawn due to concerns about increased QTc values.

64. B Lower natural killer cell activity

There is evidence to suggest immune changes in depression. There is decreased proliferation of lymphocytes in response to mitogens. In addition, the activity of natural killer cells is reduced. There are increased positive acute phase reactants and increased cytokines levels due to immune stimulation. Increased cytokines induce tryptophan oxygenase, which reduces tryptophan and hence increases the risk of depression.

65. B Transcription, modifications of mRNA, translation and finally post-translational modifications of protein into its mature form

The first step in the formation of proteins starts from transcription of DNA to RNA. RNA is then spliced to form messenger RNA (mRNA). These mRNAs are further modified and edited. Messenger RNAs are used as a template in the production of amino acids, which in turn form proteins. The translation of mRNAs to proteins is finally done with the help of transfer RNAs (tRNAs).

66. D Prevalance is 5.2:10,000 live births

Fetal alcohol syndrome is one of the common preventable causes of learning disability. One or more drink (one drink = 1.5 oz distilled spirits, 5 oz wine or 12 oz beer) per day in pregnancy increases the risk of growth retardation, which is both prenatal and postnatal. Characteristic facial features include dysmorphic facial features (flat philtrum and midface, thin upper lip along with small palpebral fissures). There is a clear dysfunction of the central nervous system, i.e. behavioural, neurological and cognitive disabilities. Prevalence of fetal alcohol syndrome is 5.2:10,000 live births.

Monozygotic twins have a concordance rate of 100% whereas it is 60–65% in dizygotic twins. There is microcephaly with irritability, inattention and poor concentration. The child will also have poor abstract reasoning along with poor executive functioning. It has been an adaptive behaviour present with major problems. Alcohol should be avoided altogether because there is no safe dose of alcohol in pregnancy though it does more harm if taken in the earlier weeks of pregnancy.

67. A Monoamine oxidase inhibitors

Narcolepsy is conventionally treated by a low dose of amphetamine and/or monoamine oxidase inhibitors. Both of these prolong the action of noradrenaline released by the nucleus ceruleus and reduce rapid eye movement sleep.

68. C γ-Aminobutyric acid

C-fos is a protein in the human body, which is encoded by the c-fos gene. It has been measured by researchers to examine neural activity in the brain. An increase in c-fos messenger RNA in the brain is indirect indication of increased neural activity. Various stimuli and neuro transmitters can activate c-fos. γ-Aminobutyric acid and glycine do not activate c-fos. Glutamate, dopamine, serotonin, noradrenaline and adrenaline, acetylcholine, antihistamine and drugs such as amphetamines, cocaine, haloperidol, morphine and caffeine activate c-fos transcription.

69. E Synapsis

During the prophase stage of meiotic division homologous chromosomes pair and come close together. This process is called pairing, which is important for recombination of genetic material.

70. C Huntington's disease

This is inherited in autosomal dominant manner. The gene responsible is an expanded and unstable CAG repeat on the short arm of chromosome 4. The onset of the disease is usually between age 30 and 50 years. People who have adult-onset Huntington's disease have CAG expansion of 40–55 repeats whereas people with childhood-onset Huntington's disease have more than 70 repeats.

71. E Lofepramine

Tricyclic antidepressants can cause ventricular arrhythmias due to blockade of cardiac sodium channels and the effect on potassium channels. Electrocardiography changes include a prolonged PR interval, QTc prolongation and unmasking of Brugada's syndrome. Lofepramine lacks arrhythmogenicity for unknown reasons.

72. D Subacute combined degeneration of the spinal cord

Vitamin B_{12} (cyanocobalamin) deficiency: subacute combined degeneration of spinal cord

Nicotinic acid: pellagra

Thiamine: Wernicke's encephalopathy

Vitamin E: peripheral and cranial nerve problems.

73. C Patau's syndrome

Edwards' syndrome results from trisomy of chromosome 18. It is characterised by severe learning disability rocker-bottom feet, low-set ears, small jaw, congenital heart disease, clenched hands and prominent occiput. Death often occurs within a year of birth.

Patau's syndrome is due to trisomy of chromosome 13. It is characterised by severe learning disability, microphthalmia, microcephaly, cleft lip or palate, abnormal forebrain structure and congenital heart disease.

74. C Metachromatic leukodystrophy: arylsulphatase A deficiency

Gaucher's disease: glucocerebrosidase deficiency

Hurler's disease: α_1-iduronidase deficiency

Niemann–Pick disease: sphingomyelinase deficiency

Tay–Sachs disease: hexosaminidase deficiency.

75. D Epistasis

This is a genetic concept. When two genes from different loci interact, they can influence a single phenotype. Mendel's concept concerned alleles that are alternative forms of genes in the same locus. One could be dominant and the other recessive. In epistasis the genes from different loci interact either resulting, or not resulting, in a single phenotype.

76. D Romano–Ward syndrome

This is an autosomal dominant genetic disorder. It is associated with a prolonged QTc interval. Ventricular arrhythmias can also be seen in the disorder. Jervell's and Lange–Nielsen syndromes also present with a prolonged QTc interval and ventricular arrhythmias; however, unlike the Romano–Ward syndrome, it also presents with congenital deafness and is an autosomal recessive disorder. DiGeorge's syndrome is a congenital immunodeficiency disorder. Characteristic signs and symptoms include congenital heart defects, raised parathyroid levels, reduced calcium levels, increased risk of infections and abnormal facies. Dressler's syndrome is inflammation of the pericardium, which occurs secondary to any injury to the heart, such as myocardial infarction or cardiac surgery. The main signs and symptoms include chest pains, joint pains, fever, pericardial and pleural effusions, and pleurisy. Brugada's syndrome is a cardiac ion channelopathy characterised by ST elevation and ventricular tachycardia. Wolfe–Parkinson–White syndrome is characterised by delta waves on ECG.

77. D M phase

Cell division consists of mitosis and meiosis. Many of the somatic cells go through cell division via the process of mitosis. Mitosis consists of the following stages: (1) interphase, (2) prophase, (3) metaphase, (4) anaphase and (5) telophase. For replication and nucleic acid synthesis each cell goes through a natural cycle called the cell cycle. The cell cycle consists of the G1 phase, S phase, G2 phase and M phase. M phase stands for mitosis phase. Division of the cell takes place in mitosis phase.

78. A Compulsive eating is limited to specific foods/ eatables/drinks

Prader–Willi syndrome occurs in 1:10,000 to 1:22,000 livebirths. It occurs due to paternal deletion of 15q11–q13 or maternal uniparental disomy of chromosome 15 or imprinting centre mutation. Hypogonadism is most useful in diagnosis during and after adolescence. Compulsive eating (hyperphagia) is the most disabling behaviour. Skin picking, found in around 20%, is the most common form of self-injury.

This syndrome is characterised by obesity, cryptorchidism, short stature, hypogonadism and hyperphagia. The lifespan depends on controlling hyperphagia. There are various food-related behaviours in Prader–Willi syndrome which include food stealing, foraging for food, gorging and indiscriminate eating.

Prader–Willi syndrome (paternal chromosome) and Angelman's syndrome (maternal chromosome) involve genes that are located in the same region in the genome and are characterised by genetic (genomic) imprinting.

79. C Abnormalities of the autosomal chromosomes usually cause severe learning disability with widespread anatomical deformities

Sex chromosomes abnormalities are not always associated with learning disabilities (LDs). Chromosomal deletions such as the cri-du-chat (cat cry) syndrome (deletion on chromosome 5), Prader–Willi syndrome (deletion on chromosome 15), 22q11.2 deletion syndrome, which has deletion on chromosome 22 and Wolf–Hirschhorn syndrome (deletion on chromosome 4) are always associated with LDs.

80. D Dentate gyrus

Basal ganglia consist of corpus striatum, amygdala and claustrum. The lentiform nucleus contains globus pallidus and putamen. The fibres responsible for the afferent connection of the hippocampus originate from the cingulate gyrus, dentate gyrus, indusium griseum (or supracallosal gyrus), parahippocampal gyrus, secondary olfactory area and septal nucleus.

81. E Von Recklinghausen's neurofibromatosis

Von Recklinghausen's neurofibromatosis: café-au-lait spots, Lisch nodules in the iris, cutaneous neurofibromas, intracranial tumours and learning disability.

Tuberous sclerosis: shagreen patch, subungual angiomas.

Sturge–Weber syndrome: strawberry naevus, port wine stain, angiomatous malformation of meningeal vessels, learning disability and epilepsy

Von Hippel-Lindau disease: vascular malformation of retina, hemangioblastoma, pancreatic, adrenal and renal cysts, and tumours.

82. D Variant CJD has an earlier onset of illness than sCJD

EEG and cerebrospinal fluid examinations are not useful in diagnosing variant CJD. Sporadic CJD is the more common of the two. The other differences are as shown in **Table 5.4**.

Table 5.4 Sporadic Creutzfeldt–Jakob disease (CJD) and variant CJD		
	Sporadic CJD	**Variant CJD**
Age of onset	55–70 years	Usually younger age. Second to fourth decades
Median duration to death	4 months	14 months
Clinical features	Rapidly progressive dementia, early change in behaviour, visual symptoms and cerebellar signs	Initial symptoms are psychiatric, mainly anxiety and depression. Limb pain and tingling, delayed cognitive difficulties with varied neurological signs
Electroencephalography	1- to 2-second triphasic waves	No characteristic signs
MRI	No characteristic sign	Pulvinar sign–high signal intensity in the pulvinar nucleus
Tonsil biopsy	Not used as a confirmatory test	Used as a confirmatory test. Scrapie prion protein (PrPSc) is found in lymphoid tissue

83. C Hypoglossal nerve

The cranial nerve, which supplies trapezius and sternocleidomastoid, is an accessory nerve. The nerve that supplies the intrinsic muscles of the tongue is the hypoglossal nerve. It is also responsible for supplying styloglossus, hyoglossus and genioglossus. The cranial nerve supplying the intrinsic muscles of the larynx is the vagus nerve. It is also responsible for supplying the constrictor muscles of the pharynx.

84. D Robertsonian translocation

This was first described in 1916 in grasshoppers. These translocations in chromosomes were named after the biologist William Robertson who first described them. Many translocations can happen across chromosomes but most of these are not compatible with life. The ones that can be seen in patients are those that involve chromosomes 13, 14, 15, 21 and 22. During robertsonian translocations (**Figure 5.1**), the centromeres of two chromosomes fuse and this leads to loss of the short arms of the chromosomes. Disorders such as Down's syndrome (trisomy 21) and Patau's syndrome (trisomy 13) can occur due to such translocations. The incidence of such translocations is roughly 1:1000 births.

85. A Imprinting genes affect the brain structure and function

From an examination of females with Turner's syndrome, it can be concluded that the brain structure and function are affected by the imprinted genes on the sex chromosome. The single X chromosome can be derived from the maternal or paternal side. If inherited from the maternal side it affects hippocampal development and if derived paternally it influences the development of the caudate nucleus and thalamus. Imprinted genes in any imprinting disorders are involved in cognitive processes. Females with Turner's syndrome do not have any Barr body. Most females with Turner's syndrome have normal intelligence.

86. C c-fos

This acts as a third messenger and can be activated by various second messengers. c-fos has been identified as an indirect measure of neural activity. Calcium, protein kinase, cAMP, phosphoinositol and arachidonic acid can act as second messengers. Calcium can also act as the first messenger. Most serotonin receptors activate a second messenger cascade.

87. B Haemangioblastomas

The following cerebral tumours are arranged in relative frequency of occurrence: gliomas, metastases, meningeal tumours, pituitary adenomas, neurilemmomas, haemangioblastomas and medulloblastomas.

Haemangioblastomas are derived from blood vessels. Gliomas are the most commonly occurring cerebral tumours.

88. E Visual association cortex

The fibres responsible for afferent connections of the hippocampus originate from the cingulate gyrus, dentate gyrus, indusium griseum, parahippocampal gyrus, secondary olfactory area and septal nucleus. The occipital lobe consists of primary visual cortex and visual association cortex.

89. E Presence of lipid peroxidation byproduct in blood

No significant difference is found in patients with and those without tardive dyskinesia with respect to cerebrospinal fluid (CSF), plasma or urinary homovanillic acid. Blood biochemistry assays have also not shown any consistent significant difference with respect to prolactin and somatotrophin. There is a role for free radical-induced neurotoxicity in the development of tardive dyskinesia. Some studies found increased blood and CSF level of lipid peroxidation.

90. D Superior mesial region

The frontal lobe consists of frontal operculum, superior medial region, inferior mesial region and dorsolateral prefrontal cortex. Frontal operculum consists of areas 44, 45 and 47. It contains Broca's area. The superior mesial region consists of a supplementary motor area and anterior cingulate cortex.

91. D Pathological crying

Emotional incontinence or pathological crying is found in post-stroke patients. The rest of the symptoms or signs are seen in temporal lobe epilepsy. In patients with temporal lobe epilepsy, they may experience an aura in which they think on a certain restricted topic and may have intrusion of stereotyped thoughts, which is called evocation of thoughts. Patients may experience thought block. They recall expansive memories in great details similar to a video clip. It is called panoramic memory. Dream-like reminiscences and altered consciousness, called uncinate crisis, have also been reported. Patients may also experience micropsia, macropsia, déjà-vu, jamais-vu, depersonalisation, gustatory hallucinations and olfactory sensations.

92. D Path analysis

This was introduced as a technique to explain the interrelations hips of variables by analysing their correlational structure and evaluating the relative importance of varying causes that influence a certain variable.

93. B Halstead–Reitan battery test

Bender's visual motor gestalt test is a perception test, which is used to evaluate visual and motor ability through the reproduction of designs. The Halstead–Reitan battery is used to detect and localise brain lesions and determine their effects. The Luria–Nebraska neuropsychological battery is used to determine left or right cerebral dominance. It is also used to identify specific types of brain dysfunction such as dyslexia. The Cambridge neuropsychological test automated battery (CANTAB) is a sensitive and specific cognitive assessment. The Wechsler's adult intelligence scale (WAIS) is a well-standardised test, which gives both verbal and performance IQ.

94. C Prophase I

In prophase 1 of meiosis, there is an alignment and contact of homologous chromosomes pairs. This allows genetic information to cross over between adjacent chromatids.

95. B Contains approximately 3.9×10^9 base-pairs

The total DNA complement in a cell is called a gene. The total DNA complement in a cell is referred to as a genome. A human DNA is more than 2 metres long. It contains approximately 3.9×10^9 base-pairs. Only 2–3% of the genome has the coding sequence of approximately 30,000 genes. The remaining part of the genome has no apparent function.

96. C 3000

In mammalian chromosome replication, approximately 3000 nucleotides are added per minute with an estimated frequency of 99.98 %.

97. A Ambivalent statements and coprolalia are characteristic features

The Lesch–Nyhan disorder is an inherited X-linked recessive disorder. It is almost entirely found in males and is extremely rare in females. The father of an affected male will neither have the disease nor be the carrier. It is an inborn error of purine nucleotide metabolism. A language that consists of ambivalent statements and coprolalia is characteristic. There is deficiency of hypoxanthine–guanine phosphoribosyltransferase (HPRT) causing hyperuricaemia. The risk to siblings depends on the carrier status of the mother. Carrier mothers have a 50% chance of transmitting the HPRT1 mutation in each pregnancy. The HPRT-encoding gene is located on the X chromosome. Self-injurious behaviour is a major behavioural presentation and involves asymmetrical compulsive self-biting, mainly of the fingers, mouth and buccal mucosa. The patient may be compulsively aggressive to others (pinching, grabbing or verbal) but will immediately apologise, admitting that behaviour was out of his control. There is a mild-to-moderate degree of learning difficulty. There are structural brain changes seen in the basal ganglia.

98. D Orexin

In animal experiments, it is found that the tuberomammillary nucleus projects widely to the cerebral cortex and maintains the awake state by activating H_1-receptors on cortical neurons. Orexin receptors are normally present on the histaminergic neurons of the tuberomammillary nucleus. The key problem is failure of production of the excitatory peptide orexin by a group of neurons in the lateral hypothalamus.

99. D Superior mesial region

The frontal lobe consists of the frontal operculum, superior mesial region, inferior mesial region and dorsolateral prefrontal cortex. The frontal operculum consists of areas 44, 45 and 47. It contains Broca's area. The superior mesial region consists of supplementary motor area and the anterior cingulate cortex.

100. D Schizophrenia

The dopamine metabolite homovanillic acid level is increased in schizophrenia and other conditions involving psychosis. It is decreased in Parkinson's disease and patients treated with antipsychotic medications. The noradrenaline metabolite vanillylmandelic acid is increased in an adrenomedullary tumour such as a phaeochromocytoma. The noradrenaline derivative metabolite, 3-methoxy-4-hydroxyphenylglycol (MHPG) 5-hydroxyindoleacetic acid (5-HIAA) is decreased in severe depression and attempted suicide.

101. A Alzheimer's dementia: diffuse slowing of α rhythm

Patients with Alzheimer's disease tend to show a slowing of α activity. As the disease progresses, α activity disappears and the EEG is dominated by θ and δ activity. The abnormality is mainly diffuse but in some cases may show predominance over the frontal and temporal lobes. Patients with frontotemporal dementia usually have a normal EEG. However, the EEG is not a reliable discriminator between frontotemporal lobe and Alzheimer's dementia, in either early or late stages. Patients with Lewy body dementia tend to show greater degree of general slowing and some more focal slow activity in the temporal region compared with those with Alzheimer's dementia. Patients with vascular dementia have α rhythm preserved for longer than those with Alzheimer's dementia. In some cases, there may be intermittent slow activity in the temporal lobes. It is not surprising that patients with pseudodementia have a normal EEG tracing. In Huntington's disease/dementia there is low-voltage EEG, initial loss of α waves and later a flattened EEG trace.

102. C Mitochondria

DNA is mainly contained in the cell nucleus. A tiny amount of DNA is also present in mitochondria. In a fertilised egg, mitochondria are mainly derived from the mother's side so inheritance of mitochondria is mainly through the female lineage. Mitochondrial disorders are usually responsible for degenerative disorders including ageing. As transmission of mitochondrial DNA is mother to child, it can be used for genealogical research into an individual's maternal side.

103. B Bradford Hill criteria

These criteria are still widely accepted in the modern era, as a logical structure for investigating and defining causality in an epidemiological study. The criteria are: consistency, specificity, temporality, and plausibility, strength of association, biological gradient, coherence, reversibility and analogy.

104. C Positional cloning

The association between Alzheimer's disease and Down's syndrome helps in the detection of linkage of familial Alzheimer's disease on chromosome 21, and is known as positional cloning; it is also sometimes called 'reverse genetics'. It is a method of gene identification. A gene, the candidate gene, is identified for a specific phenotype (which will be Down's syndrome in this case) in the region (candidate region), and other common traits due to this candidate region. This is followed by positional cloning which basically involves identification of DNA segments that overlap along the chromosome towards a candidate gene. The candidate gene approach states that a major component of variation of a phenotype under investigation might be caused by polymorphism of the candidate gene.

105. C Post-translational processing

Gene expression is mainly controlled at the level of transcription, although translational control and post-translational processing might be important for some genes. DNA methylation causes gene inactivation by adding methyl groups to cytosine bases.

106. A Congenital heart malformations are present in 50% of patients with Down's syndrome

In 1887, Down gave the first description of Down's syndrome. The underlying genetic abnormality (trisomy 21) was identified in 1959. Down's syndrome was the first syndrome in which the typical physical features were related to a chromosomal anomaly. It accounts for a third of the children in special education. Life expectancy is less, especially due to the congenital heart malformation. Hypotonia and short stature are typical. The hypotonia becomes less apparent as the individuals grow up. Fifteen per cent are hypothyroid by adolescence. Heart malformations are present in 50%. Approximately 7% have congenital upper intestinal obstructions, and 1% have a diagnosis of leukaemia. Hearing impairment occurs in 60–80% along with visual problems and delayed bone maturation.

107. C Pleiotropism

Pleiotropy is from the Greek *pleio*, which means many, and *tropic*, which means affecting. Mutation of a single gene can give rise to a disease with multiple unrelated phenotypes; an example in humans is phenylketonuria. Mutation of the PAH gene results in reduced/absent activity of phenylalanine hydroxylase. This can lead to learning difficulties, eczema and pigmentary changes in the skin.

108. D High risk for dementia in adults with Down's syndrome has been linked to triplication and overexpression of the gene for amyloid precursor protein

There is early onset of menopause and dementia in women with Down's syndrome. Evidence of dementia is found in up to half of the patients after age 50. In Down's syndrome, there is triplication and overexpression of the gene for amyloid precursor protein (APP). Alzheimer-type dementia is the most common dementia in patients with Down's syndrome. The neuropathological changes are more commonly seen before behavioural manifestations and may be misleading. The ε2 allele is protective; an ε4 homozygote is associated with increased risk. In Down's syndrome, women with early menopause (46 years of age or younger) were found to have earlier onset and increased risk of Alzheimer's disease compared with woman who have their menopause after age 46. It is the bioavailabili rather than the total estradio that is associated with dementia.

109. C Metaphase stage of meiotic division

Cross-over of genetic material results in recombination. During the metaphase stage, chromatids of homologous chromosomes exchange segments by breakage and recombination. Usually, this happens during meiotic division. It is an important process to maintain genetic diversity. Sometimes, it can happen in mitotic division in eukaryotes when there is loss of, or damage to, a segment of chromosome. Recombination helps to repair the genetic material in this situation.

110. D Offspring of an individual with deletion of 22q11.2 syndrome have a 50% chance of inheriting the 22q11.2 deletion

This is inherited as autosomal dominant. Approximately a quarter of patients with velocardiofacial syndrome (VCSF) develop psychotic symptoms. This syndrome is denoted as 22q11.2 deletion syndrome and includes VCSF and DiGeorge's syndrome. The offspring of an individual 22q11.2 deletion syndrome have a 50% chance of inheriting the 22q11.2 deletion. The psychotic and affective symptoms sometimes do emerge in adolescence or early adulthood. Overall the prevalence of schizophrenia in VCSF is 25 times more than in the general population. The psychosis associated with VCSF usually runs a chronic course and exhibits a poor response to antipsychotic treatment. The VCSF is typically characterised by cleft palate (commonest syndrome associated with cleft palate), cardiac abnormalities and mild learning disabilities. The patient has a long face with a prominent upper jaw and flattening of his cheeks, and a small open mouth with an underdeveloped lower jaw. Hypocalcaemia and immunodeficiency are present. The 22q11 deletion syndrome (22qds) is the second most common human chromosomal anomaly after Down's syndrome (trisomy 21) and occurs in approximately in 1: 4,000 births.

111. A 45,X

Aneuploidy usually arises from failure of pained chromosomes or sister chromatids to disjoin at anaphase (non-disjunction). Alternatively, aneuploidy may be due to delayed movement of a chromosome at anaphase (anaphase lag). Thus, by either mechanisms two cells are produced, one with an extra copy of chromosomes in trisomy and one with them missing in monosomy. The cause is unknown, but increases in incidence with maternal age.

Polyploidy is the presence of a complete extra set of chromosomes, i.e. 46 + 23 is triploidy with 69 chromosomes and 46 + 46 is tetraploidy with 96 chromosomes. The polyploid cells occur normally in human bone marrow among megakaryocytes. The tetraploid cells are also a feature of regenerating livers.

112. B 200

Lithium is available in two preparations: lithium carbonate and lithium citrate. The prophylactic prescription needs specialist advice. The initiation and change in treatment require more monitoring. The preparation differs widely in bioavailability.

The lithium content and treatment dosage depend on the preparations; 5 mL lithium citrate (520 mg/5 mL) is equivalent to 200 mg lithium carbonate.

Table 5.5 Lithium salts		
Lithium carbonate		
	Priadel 200 MR	Lithium 5.4 mmol/L
	Camcolit 250 MR	Lithium 6.8 mmol/L
	Liskonium 450 MR	Lithium 12.2 mmol/L
Lithium citrate		
	Liq Priadel 520 mg/5 mL	Lithium 5.4 mmol/L

113. C Incidence

This is the new occurrence over a period of time of a disease. Prevalence is the total number of new and old existing cases of that disease at that time. Both are routinely standardised for easy inference.

114. D Regulating function of dopamine in the frontal cortex

Dysbindin (DTNBP1) affects glutamate release. Neuregulin (NRG1) plays a role in brain development, synaptic plasticity and glutamate signalling. COMT is involved in dopamine regulation in frontal cortex. G72 (DAOA) affects the metabolism of the NMDA-receptor modulator D-serine. Disrupted in schizophrenia 1 (DISC1) contributes via its role in brain development, cell functioning and synaptic signalling. PPP3CC has an important role in integration of dopamine and glutamate signalling.

115. A Down's syndrome

Senile plaques are seen in ageing and Down's syndrome. Neurofibrillary tangles are seen in Down's syndrome, ageing, dementia pugilistic (chronic traumatic encephalopathy), Lytico–Bodig disease (progressive paralysis resembling amyotrophic lateral sclerosis), postencephalitic Parkinson's disease, and progressive supranuclear palsy.

116. A Cingulate gyrus

Along with the cingulate gyrus, the prefrontal cortex motor cortex, primary auditory cortex and supplementary motor area supply efferents to the anterior thalamic nucleus, ventral anterior nuclei, posterior part of ventral lateral thalamic nuclei, medial geniculate body and anterior part of ventral lateral thalamic nuclei.